ALL YOU NEED TO KNOW....

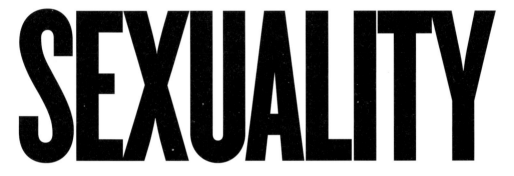

SEXUALITY

BY CHARLIE McCANN

10 9 8 7 6 5 4 3 2 1

ISBN 978-1-912568-03-1

First published as *All you need to know: Sexuality*
by Connell Publishing in 2018

Picture credits:
Cover illustration © NatBasil / Shutterstock
Harmodius © 2006 Sergey Sosnovskiy p12
Wellcome Collection © pp 16, 41, 68, 75, 95, 98, 112, 115
Alamy collection © p29

Design: Ben Brannan
Associate Publisher: Paul Woodward
Editor: Jolyon Connell
Assistant Editor and typesetter: Alfred Fletcher

Printed in Great Britain

To Simon

CONTENTS

INTRODUCTION

Humans have always had sex. But look through the keyhole of the past and you will see they have not always done it in the same manner, with the same kinds of people or with the same beliefs about whether what they are doing is right or desirable. Attitudes to sex shape what happens in the bedroom and as these attitudes shift, so does sexual behaviour. In 1936, Havelock Ellis, an English sexologist, cited the case of a respectable, married woman who was a leading campaigner for chastity.

> [She] discovered through reading some pamphlets against solitary vice, that she had herself been practicing masturbation for years without knowing it. The profound anguish and hopeless despair of this woman in the face of what she believed to be the moral ruin of her whole life cannot well be described.

She realised that what she had believed was a harmless pleasure was universally condemned across Europe and the United States as a wicked act that could lead to blindness, paralysis, insanity or even death. If only she had come to this realisation 50 years later, when Western society's attitude towards masturbation had transformed almost beyond recognition. The solitary vice was now seen as medically benign and even celebrated for the way it put into practice the idea of pleasure for its own sake.

At its core, "sexuality" is an individual's experience of the erotic, an experience which is shaped by one's desires and relationships, sexual acts and identities. The woman from Ellis's anecdote clearly prided herself on having the sexuality of a respectable, heterosexual woman (that is, until she read those pamphlets). But what it meant to be a respectable, heterosexual woman in inter-war Britain will remain a mystery until we discover how that society understood sex.

This brings us to the other definition of "sexuality": the constellation of meanings that societies attach to sex. This constellation is formed at any given moment by a number of forces: the urge or injunction to reproduce, cultural expectations about how men and women should look and behave (also known as gender), and of course desire, that "insistent psychic energy which torments as much as it drives human action", as historian Jeffrey Weeks writes. Economic, social, religious and political forces shape sexuality, as do prevailing ideas about race, ethnicity and the biology of the body. Categories like "homosexuality" and "heterosexuality" are invented to help organise our thinking about sexuality, as we shall see.

Historians debate when, precisely, these categories were invented. Today, Western society thinks of sexuality as a fundamental component of the psyche, one that marks individuals out as particular types of people: a homosexual, heterosexual or bisexual, for instance – identities that determine not only with whom one has sex, and how, but one's lifestyle and even character. In his seminal work *The History of Sexuality*, Michel Foucault contended that this is a relatively recent phenomenon, as he argued the history of same-sex relations proves. During the medieval and early-modern eras, men who had sex with other men were punished for committing the forbidden act of sodomy. By contrast, their Victorian counterparts were penalised for belonging to a distinct sexual species: the "homosexual". This shift, from a society in which anyone could be charged with committing an illicit act, to one in which certain types of people were seen as predisposed to particular kinds of sexual behaviour, heralded the arrival of an age in which sexual identity defined the self.

Foucault's thesis has been widely debated since its first outing in 1978. Many historians have rightly pointed out that identities of people living before the 19th century were fundamentally shaped by their sexuality, just not in ways that we would recognise today. Medieval people, for instance, defined themselves according to whether they were chaste or sexually active rather than homosexual or heterosexual, as historian Ruth Mazo Karras shows. Though Foucault's historical analysis is flawed, the insight underpinning it is not. Sexuality is not a fixed, biological constant: it is shaped by society as well as by the body.

The general reader interested in exploring the ever-shifting constellation of meanings orbiting around sex in the West will find in this book a brief guide. Beginning with the world of antiquity and ending with the present, it will stop at a number of way stations: among them, the gymnasiums of ancient Greece, where men seduced boys; caves occupied by Christian ascetics who strove to snuff out their lust; the fashionable drawing rooms of Georgian London, where libertines hunted for women to prey on; and the bars of Weimar Berlin, where lesbians debated the nature of their desire. A tour as short as this must speed past destinations readers might prefer to linger over, in which case, do consult the bibliography.

CHAPTER ONE

SEX AND THE CITY: ANCIENT GREECE AND ROME

Timarchos should have known better. Having squandered his inheritance on wine, gambling, flute girls and prostitutes, he began selling his body to wealthy men in order to maintain his profligate lifestyle. That Timarchos, an adult citizen of fourth-century BC Athens, a Greek city-state, would sleep with men – and for money, no less – appalled his fellow citizens. An orator named Aeschines accused Timarchos of being morally unfit to participate in the public life of the city and took him to court. Yet during the trial, Aeschines, admitting that he had had relationships with several boys himself, hastened to point out that he had slept only with youths never with men, and reminded his audience that such liaisons were perfectly legal. Evidently, Timarchos had not scandalised Athens by sleeping with members of his own sex. He had transgressed by sleeping with grown men rather than male youths.

The sexual culture of ancient Greece and Rome was very different from our own. Statues of Priapus, the Greek god of fertility most frequently depicted with an enormous, erect phallus, guarded the gates of Athenian estates. Inside wealthy Roman homes, frescoes of copulating couples adorned living-room walls, while vases decorated with sexually explicit scenes were owned by commoners and wealthy alike. The unabashed frankness with which the Greeks and Romans incorporated erotic images into their public lives reflected their view of desire. In itself, it was nothing to be ashamed of. Desire was a powerful energy that moved through every human, just as it moved through the beasts and the gods, linking them all together in one chain of being.

Properly harnessed by reason and self-restraint, desire was regarded as a positive force. It was celebrated for ensuring the survival of civilisation at fertility festivals like Liberalia, held in honour of Roman boys who had ejaculated for the first time. Though sex was closely associated with procreation, the two were not synonymous; sex could be had for the pleasure of it, and not just between men and women. Mortals emulated Zeus, the Greek deity who openly consorted with his handsome male cupbearer, Ganymede, even though he had a wife. Not only was it acceptable for desire to flow between men; at times, it was actively encouraged. Plato, an Athenian philosopher, believed that devotion to a boy was one step on a man's journey to a nobler love of wisdom and truth. Harmodius and Aristogiton, heroes who died liberating Athens from a tyrant, were feted throughout the ancient world for their love for each other and their city.

Sometimes, though, the callous god of desire, Eros, threatened to overpower the reason of his victims by shooting one too many arrows into their hearts. That's what happened to Timarchos. His lust rendered him a slave to his pleasures. This was not how an upstanding Athenian citizen was supposed to behave. Athenian society evaluated conduct based on whether it was honourable or shameful. Men of honour disciplined their desires by exercising *enkrateia*, or self-control. In classical Athens, which had become a democracy by the fifth century BC, this quality was embodied by the hoplite. A courageous citizen-soldier, the hoplite was "stronger than himself", as a popular saying had it, because he successfully subdued his lusts for food, drink and sex. Just as the hoplite ruled victorious over his animal appetites, he was expected to control the women and slaves in his household, assert his dominance over his fellow citizens in the forum, and triumph over the Persians on the battlefield. In Athenian society, which was strictly hierarchical and relentlessly competitive, the hoplite staked his

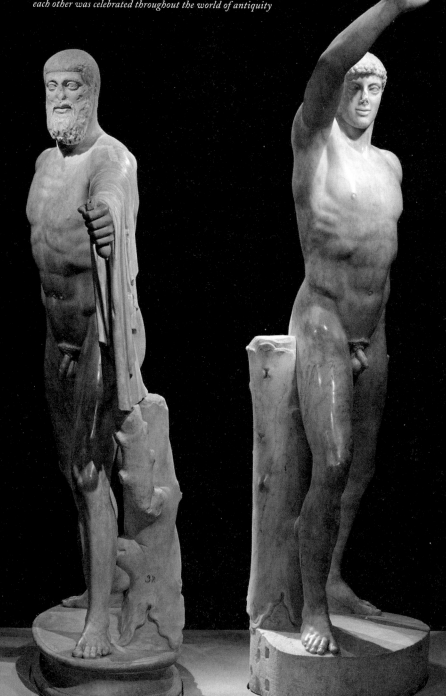

Harmodius and Aristogiton, Greek lovers whose devotion to
each other was celebrated throughout the world of antiquity

claim to status by prevailing over his social subordinates. But he could not rule over others until he could first govern himself.

This ideal of masculinity, which the Athenians shared with the Romans, shaped a man's sexual conduct. He was expected to aggressively demonstrate his superiority over others in the bedroom just as he did in the household, the forum and the battlefield. He did so by physically penetrating his social inferiors, a category that included women and non-citizen men – slaves, for instance. Because women were defined in opposition to men – they were sexually passive while men were active – it was considered normal for women to be penetrated and natural for them to enjoy it. But for a man to take pleasure in playing the passive was deeply transgressive because it meant relinquishing control of his body to another, like a woman would. In his speech denouncing Timarchos, Aeschines gravely insults him by describing him as "this man with a man's body, but who has sinned womanly sins". Effeminate men such as Timarchos represented the polar opposite of the hoplite: they were branded *kinaidoi*, men who inspired fear and revulsion because they relished being sexually penetrated.

It would be easy to assume that Timarchos was homosexual but the ancients did not think about sexual identity as we do today. In fact, sexual orientation was of minor consideration to the Greeks and Romans, who assumed that most men were interested in both men and women. Because sexual relations mirrored social relations, what mattered was not whether one's partner was male or female but whether the role one played during sex was that of the social superior or inferior. Julius Caesar was roundly mocked for his relationship with Nicomedes, king of Bithynia, not because he was sleeping with a man but because, it was rumoured, he played the passive, feminine role. In surrendering his body to a man, Caesar – like Timarchos, 300 years before him – had acted like a slave or woman, not a leader of men. As Caesar's soldiers gleefully chanted at the triumph honouring his conquest of Gaul, "Caesar conquered Gaul; Nicomedes, Caesar".

***

If Timarchos had slept with boys rather than adult men, he would not have provoked such scorn. In Athens, boys were inferior to men, so it was legally, morally and socially acceptable for the latter to have sex with the former. In fact, the literature of the period, from the dialogues of Plato to the poetry of Catullus, vaunts such love. Possessed of hairless, muscular bodies and small penises, which men regarded as erotic, teenage boys represented the pinnacle of male beauty.

Ordinary Athenians could solicit the services of prostitutes, both male and female, in the city's cheap, state-run brothels. Members of the elite engaged in pederasty, a practice in which a man struck up a sexual relationship with an aristocratic adolescent. The lover (*erastes*) met his beloved (*eromenos*) at the gymnasium, where boys exercised nude, or at symposia, exclusive drinking parties. He wooed him by giving him gifts and educating him in the ways of the world. If his advances were reciprocated the *erastes* would be permitted to consummate the relationship by inserting his penis in between the thighs or into the anus of his *eromenos*. Such relationships lasted only for as long as the beloved remained a youth. Theognis, a sixth-century BC poet from the Greek city of Megara, writes,

Boy, so long as you have a smooth cheek, I will never
stop praising, not if it is my fate to die.

But as peach fuzz gave way to bristles, the charms of the *eromenos* started to fade. As he matured into a man, acquiring the status of citizen, he would begin to court his very own beloved, starting the whole cycle over again.

The Athenian elite embraced pederasty as a way of introducing boys into the world of men but it also inspired much hand-wringing. Boys would someday need to become manly citizen-soldiers; some would even be future leaders of Athens. If they acted improperly in their youth, by surrendering too easily to the caresses of their suitors, by having multiple affairs or by enjoying penetration, they could be embarrassed as adults and public figures. As a result, beautiful Adonises from the elite – seen as particularly desirable – had to walk a "difficult tightrope of desire", as classicist Kirk Ormand observes. They couldn't throw themselves at their suitors, but neither could they turn down all their admirers. When selecting their lovers, the most virtuous youths would exercise restraint and good judgement – the very qualities they would need to be successful citizens later in life. The law afforded *eromenoi* some protection. Those who sexually violated boys, women or men were deprived of their rights as citizens.

The anxiety underpinning Athens's rules on pederasty stemmed from a broader concern about sexual passivity, one it shared with Rome. Passivity was not in itself illegal in either society but it invited opprobrium. Roman politicians were so fearful that free-born boys would come to enjoy playing the part of the passive as adults that they outlawed the kind of pederasty practised by Greeks, while in Athens, citizens suspected of passivity could be accused of prostituting themselves, which the law prohibited free men from doing. Those convicted were stripped of the rights of citizenship: they could no longer sponsor new laws, serve as an ambassador for the state, or make formal accusations against other citizens in a court of law. Allegations of prostitution could officially be made at regular public meetings in which any citizen could challenge the fitness of another to play a leading role in Athenian politics.

They often did. Aeschines, the orator, was determined to destroy Timarchos's political career, so in 345 BC he accused him of prostitution. In his speech, he portrayed Timarchos as a man who liked playing the passive. This was the ultimate insult, but Aeschines didn't stop there. He argued that a man who has sold his body and who has indulged in excessive sexual pleasures is not a man who is in control of himself. A man who cannot control his person cannot control his household and a man who cannot control his household cannot control the affairs of the city:

> And shall we send out as an ambassador of the city this man who has lived shamefully at home, and trust this man with the most important matters? What would he not give away, this man who has sold the right to abuse his body?

In this way of thinking by analogy, the personal is political: the Athenian who sells his body would not think twice about selling out the body politic. If it got the better of one's self-control, desire could turn men into traitors – to themselves and their city.

***

The risks posed to a citizen's honour were particularly pronounced when Eros set his sights on daughters and wives. Greek and Roman men idealised women who were meek, virtuous and domestic. On Greek vases, men were portrayed as bronzed by the sun but women – who were meant to stay inside the house – were pale. Yet, as historian Anna Clark observes, the female characters of Athenian drama were far from submissive: a vengeful Clytemnestra murders her husband; Lysistrata convinces the women of Athens to protest a war by denying their men sex. Playwrights like Aristophanes tapped into a male fear that women's dormant passion – held in check by what little *enkrateia* they had – would easily erupt and overwhelm them. This fear also gnawed at Roman men. The poet Catullus wailed that his fickle lover, Lesbia, "takes on three hundred lovers at once, not being truly in love with any, but breaking the groins of all."

In Greece, the belief that women were sexually insatiable and lacking in that quintessentially male virtue, *enkrateia*, justified denying them political autonomy and sequestering them at home, where they were to live removed from temptation in an exclusively female world surrounded by mothers, female relatives and servants. There, girls were trained in the domestic arts in preparation for marriage, the primary purpose of which was the production of legitimate heirs. To that end, fathers arranged matches for

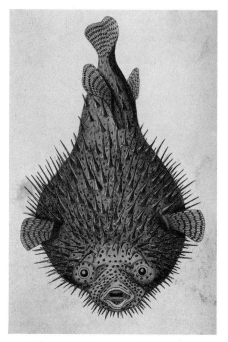

Husbands took revenge on the lovers of their wives by sticking spiky things like this fish up their anuses

their daughters while they were still teenagers, fearing for their daughters' virtue if they weren't promptly married off. If a father found out that his unmarried daughter was pregnant, he could sell her into slavery.

Once wedded, wives were to remain devoted to their husbands. A wife's infidelity was a serious crime, for it not only dishonoured her husband, it also threw into question the legitimacy of offspring. The repercussions were severe. In Rome, a husband could abandon his infant if he did not want to acknowledge it as his own, while in Athens, a man who knew his wife was unfaithful was required to divorce her. Failure to do so amounted to an admission that she was a prostitute and he a pimp. Both societies permitted husbands to rape and kill their wives' lovers, if caught in the act.

While female virtue was sacrosanct, no laws prevented a husband from sleeping around and there was little disapproval of such behaviour on moral grounds. One Roman writer thought it sufficient to restrain male fidelity "to the walls around the house, not to tie it down to the marriage bed itself." Slaves and servants were fair game, and Greek and Roman men commonly solicited the services of prostitutes and high-class courtesans. As Apollodorus, an Athenian politician, noted, "we have courtesans for pleasure, and concubines for the daily service of our bodies, [and] wives for the production of legitimate offspring and to have a reliable guardian of our household property."

Some wives would have scoffed at men like Apollodorus. They couldn't all be as silent and obedient as the women decorating Greek vases. In Aristophanes's comedy, *Lysistrata*, the eponymous heroine declares, "A man never enjoys himself unless it suits his wife." Though this line is clearly an exaggeration, it wouldn't have amused Aristophanes's male audience if the idea that wives were manipulating men like marionettes didn't ring true. It suggests that some women, at least, wielded influence over their husbands.

Roman men had more cause to be uneasy about female power than the Greeks. Though Roman women were legally the wards of a male guardian, they enjoyed greater freedoms than their Greek sisters. They could go out to dinner and attend the theatre as long as they were accompanied by their husbands. Women could legally own property, divorce their husbands for abysmal behaviour (like bringing a mistress back home), and acquire prestige as patrons of artists and writers. These freedoms had the effect of "making the wife a partner of her husband, not a ward," as classicist Kyle Harper writes. The elite hoped that, though marriages were arranged, love and friendship would blossom in such partnerships. Some Romans whispered, however, that women were taking advantage of this liberal climate to commit adultery. Julia, the daughter of Augustus, the first Roman Emperor, allegedly took many lovers. The consequences of breaching society's expectations of her sex were serious. Eventually Julia was found out, convicted of adultery, and exiled by her father.

***

What the men and women of antiquity did together behind closed doors is shrouded in mystery. But just as the Romans illuminated their bedrooms with lamps decorated with the winged figure of Eros, classicists have been able to cast some light on ancient sexual practices. Men regarded women as sexual objects to be penetrated, in the vagina, anus or mouth – all points of entry were considered acceptable and normal, though fellatio was seen as an act performed by prostitutes rather than wives. Cunnilingus was regarded with disgust, which goes to show how little women's pleasure mattered. Yet the widespread belief that women would conceive only if they orgasmed suggests that husbands would have tried to satisfy their wives. This idea contributed to a Roman literature celebrating mutual pleasure between husband and wife. According to Harper, the female orgasm was actually discussed more during the Roman Empire than it ever had been before or would be for centuries after.

The belief that conception depended on mutual orgasm was spread by doctors. Philo, a philosopher from the first century, articulated the prevailing medical view when he said, "Apart from pleasure nothing of mortal kind comes into existence." Most physicians believed that orgasm was a sign that the womb had drawn up male and female ejaculate and closed itself off. To ensure that the womb received this mixture, physicians encouraged husbands to satisfy their wives.

This understanding of reproductive biology belonged to a theory of the body which held that women had the same basic anatomy as men (which explains why women were believed to produce semen). As historian Thomas Laqueur has shown, many experts believed that the vagina and ovaries were essentially a penis and testicles, except that, as Nemesius, a fourth-century bishop, put it, "theirs are inside the body and not outside it." Galen, the pre-eminent anatomist of the age, thought that women retained these organs inside their bodies because they had less vital heat, the substance animating the human body, than men. This distinction was important – it was seen as an expression of man's superiority – but it was a difference of degree rather than kind. Unlike Aristotle, who argued that there were two radically distinct sexes, Galen believed that there was just one sex. Men were the perfect expression of this basic body type while women, with their undescended penises, were less developed and less perfect. This theory would remain influential until the late 18th century.

***

Did the women of antiquity have erotic experiences independently of men? It is hard to say. Greek and Roman literature was, by and large, written by men, about men, for men. When men wrote about women, it was typically in relation to their own lives. There is so little evidence for sexual relations between Athenian women, for instance, that one scholar has surmised that it amounts to a conspiracy of silence on the part of the Athenians.

Yet a few clues do exist. In a poem by Herondas, a Greek poet from the second century BC, two women discuss a friend's strap-on dildo. So delightful is this length of leather that several women have borrowed it. Not only does this poem reveal that "dildos travel", as Ormand observes, it suggests that a tight-knit society of women "who literally share sexual experiences" existed. Another hint can be found in the poetry of Sappho, a sixth-century BC poet from the island of Lesbos and the only surviving female voice from this period. In the fragments that remain of her fervid poetry, love – "the limb-loosener" – wracks women who are consumed with unrequited love for each other.

Many centuries later, the Romans would describe Sappho as a *tribas*. This term emerged in the second century AD as an insult for a woman who was considered masculine because she played the active role during sex, typically with other women. (Some *tribades* were even thought to possess large clitorises which, it was suggested, permitted them to sexually penetrate their conquests.) The existence of this term suggests that some Roman women, at least, were known for having sex with other women.

But just as Greek and Roman men who slept with each other should not be seen as homosexuals, *tribades* should not be seen as lesbians. There is no evidence to suggest that they identified as women exclusively attracted to other women, or that that was why they attracted such censure. They were shamed not for their choice of partner but for the masculine manner in which they disported themselves. Gender norms dictated the sexual behaviour of the ancients: men proved they were men by sexually dominating their subordinates, while women were defined by the pleasure they took in being dominated. *Tribades* violated these expectations by playing the part of the man. This sexual value system would eventually be challenged by the champions of an upstart new religion from a far-flung corner of the Roman Empire: Palestine.

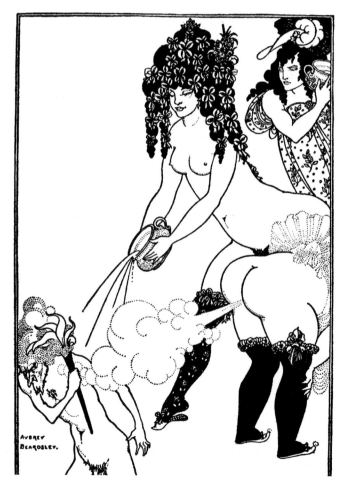

A scene from Aristophanes's play Lysistrata *entitled* Lysistrata Defending the Acropolis *(1896) by Aubrey Beardsley*

CHAPTER TWO

EXTRA VIRGIN: EARLY CHRISTIANITY

In the second half of the first century AD, a wealthy young man from a Roman city in modern-day Turkey brought a complaint to the local governor. Thamyris was bitterly angry, for his beautiful fiancé, Thecla, had been seduced by the words of a wandering preacher named Paul. His sermons, about the teachings of a man named Jesus, entreated those who would follow the Christian God to abandon marriage and embrace celibacy. Captivated, Thecla promised to break off her engagement and remain a virgin forever. In an audience with the governor, Thamyris bitterly condemned Paul:

> This man has introduced a new teaching, bizarre and disruptive of the human race. He denigrates marriage: yes, marriage, which you might say is the beginning, root and fountainhead of our nature. From it spring fathers, mothers, children and families. Cities, villages and cultivation have appeared because of it. Agriculture,

the sailing of the seas and all the skills of this state...depend on it. What is more, from marriage come the temples and sanctuaries of our land, sacrifice, rituals, initiations, prayers and solemn days of intercession.

This paean to marriage and marital sex was not the hyperbole of a lovelorn suitor. For all its prosperity, Roman society was "grazed thin by death". When the empire was at its height in the second century AD, the average life expectancy was less than 25 years. Spurred on by custom and legislation punishing bachelors and rewarding couples who had children, men and women did their part to replace the dead. (The pressure on women would have been enormous: for the population of the empire to remain stable, every woman had to give birth to an average of five children.) But Thamyris's appeals, to tradition and the survival of the community, failed to move Thecla. Tossed into prison, where she joined Paul, she eventually escaped, and would over the years risk rape, torture and execution in order to remain a virgin devoted to God.

The struggle between Thamyris, champion of Roman family values, and Thecla, bride of Christ, encapsulates a conflict that would roil the empire as Jesus of Nazareth's message spread, slowly at first, from the groves of Galilee where he first preached, then with speed, as his disciples fanned out across the empire to proclaim the Word of God. The Christian movement condemned what it saw as the hedonism of pagan sexual culture and vaunted the virtues of virginity and chastity. This arose from a new understanding of sexual desire that was fundamentally at odds with the pagan view. To the Greeks and Romans, the sex drive was a manifestation of the energy that pulsed through the cosmos, linking humans to animals and the stars. Like all the passions, lust needed to be bridled, but it was also a necessary expression of humanity's connection to nature. The Christian view was diametrically opposed. As Clement of Alexandria, a second-century theologian, succinctly put it:

Man's capacity for continence, as far as the Greek philosophers regard it, is said to be a matter of striving against desire...The Christian ideal is not to experience desire at all.

Lust did not merely test one's self-control. To Christians it sullied the soul, for desire was the Devil's handmaiden. By inspiring Eve to seduce Adam, it brought about the very first sin and the punishment for it: mankind's fall from grace. This reading of the Biblical story of creation fixed desire at the centre of a cosmic battle between good and evil. Whenever lust stirred the groins of Adam and Eve's descendants, the Devil was inviting them to sin once again. Those who could extinguish desire scored a victory for God.

This view of desire as inherently wicked was the keystone of a Christian sexual ethics that the early leaders of the Church had started to erect. Their moral code idealising virginity and forbidding almost all sex, unless it was for the purpose of procreation, would bring about a "revolution in sexual attitudes and practises", according to historian Elaine Pagels. As Christianity grew from a small movement – one of many new faiths jostling for attention in late antiquity – to become the official religion of the Roman Empire in 380, Thecla would, according to her legend, topple Venus from her pedestal as if she were a "wanton maid" and banish her from the empire.

***

In the first days of Christianity, it was not a given that sex and desire would be regarded with horror. The Jewish tradition from which Christianity sprang celebrated marital sex and fertility and Jesus himself praised monogamous marriage as a renewal of the bond uniting Adam and Eve. He did not, however, count consistency among his virtues: though Jesus said that marriage was blessed by God, he also called those who remained unmarried "equal to angels" and praised those "who made themselves eunuchs for the sake of the kingdom of heaven". (Origen, a third-century theologian, took Jesus at his word and castrated himself. Few were inspired to follow suit.) The life of Jesus was more instructive in this respect than his words. He was believed to have been unmarried and chaste. The Church Fathers took note.

The man who converted Thecla contributed far more to the fashioning of a Christian sexual morality than Jesus. Paul the Apostle was the first of Jesus's followers to translate his teachings into practical advice about sexual behaviour. A tent maker who journeyed through the Roman world a few decades after Jesus's death, he informed his converts that the body was a "temple of the Holy Spirit"; it therefore needed to remain pure. Sex was polluting. This echoed the old Jewish belief that sex was unclean, but unlike the Jews, who revered marital intercourse (as long as husband and wife bathed afterwards), Paul urged his followers to abstain from sex. Jesus was expected to return to Earth at any moment to judge the living and the dead. With the end of the world approaching, the faithful could ill afford to be distracted by worldly matters like marriage and mewling babies. They needed to attend to their souls.

Paul did concede, though, that some would be too weak to be celibate, as he was. For such people "it is better to marry than to burn". Paul did not regard marital sex, with its potential for procreation, as positive in itself – the Second Coming was nigh and the propagation of mankind unnecessary. But he acknowledged that marital sex would discourage Christians who struggled with desire from committing the sin of adultery.

This was a grudging toleration of marital sex only. On no account were Christians to behave like the lecherous pagans. Paul proclaimed that "neither fornicators, nor idolaters, nor adulterers, nor the effeminate, nor men who have sex with men" would be admitted to the kingdom of heaven. Paul did not look kindly on the sexual freedoms permitted to men in Greek and Roman society. For him, all "fornication", or extra-marital sex, was shameful, no matter whether committed by a man or a woman, by the active or the passive. He hoped that sexual purity would set Christians apart from the sinful pagan world.

***

From the outset, then, the Church was conflicted about sex. On the one hand, it idealised chastity; on the other, it acknowledged that abstinence was hard. In the centuries following Paul's death in around 60 AD, one camp seemed to gain the upper hand. An influential movement of radical Christians claimed that all sex was sinful, even marital sex. After all, they said, God had thrown Adam and Eve out of Eden for acquiring carnal knowledge of each other. Ascetics retreated to the deserts of Egypt where they confronted the very temptations to which Adam and Eve had succumbed. They believed that if they could quell the desires of the flesh, for food, sex and companionship, they could succeed where Adam had not.

Celibacy was by no means unheard of at the time. Stoic philosophers encouraged Greek and Roman men to rein in their lust. From the second century BC, colonies of Jewish men in Palestine permanently abstained from sex. But these movements belonged to the fringes of their cultures, which on the whole promoted marriage and family. By contrast, ascetics – both male and female – belonged to the Christian mainstream. Stories of their heroic acts of renunciation became wildly popular. As a young man, St Anthony gave his money to the poor and retreated to the barren wastes of the Egyptian desert, where he prayed, fasted and tried to dispel the visions of beautiful women the Devil tempted him with.

Virtually all Christians agreed that the ascetic was closer to the kingdom of heaven than the married householder. But by the fourth century, as the prospect of the Second Coming of Christ became increasingly remote, the Church Fathers began to consider the long-term future of the religion. If it were to survive and grow, marriages and households would be necessary. They began to argue that the ascetics went too far when they said that sex was always sinful: all of God's creation was good, even the body, for hadn't the Son of God assumed physical form? And hadn't God commanded humans to "go forth and multiply"? Though the married Christian could never shine as brightly as "the most brilliant stars" in the kingdom of heaven – the virgins – there was a place for him in the firmament.

The Church Fathers hastened to add that this did not mean that married couples could yield to desire for each other. They could have sex as long as it remained untainted by passion. This rather tortured policy derived from Clement of Alexandria's interpretation of the story of Adam and Eve. He believed that God had evicted them from paradise not because they had sex, but because they had sex too soon. They gave in to their lust for each other without first securing God's blessing. According to this analysis, desire was to blame for the fall of mankind, not sex.

To minimise the chances that Christians might repeat Adam and Eve's mistake, Clement decreed that sex was only permissible for the purpose of reproduction. All sexual acts that could not result in conception were forbidden: among them, oral and anal sex, intercourse with a wife who was menstruating, pregnant, menopausal or barren, and mystifyingly sex in the morning, in the daytime or after dinner. Embracing one's wife for the pleasure of it was, of course, a mortal sin. "A man who is too passionately in love with his wife is an adulterer," said Jerome, a fourth-century theologian. Once the Christian couple had fulfilled their obligation to be fruitful and

25

The Temptation of St Anthony *(c.1650)*,
by Joos van Craesbeeck

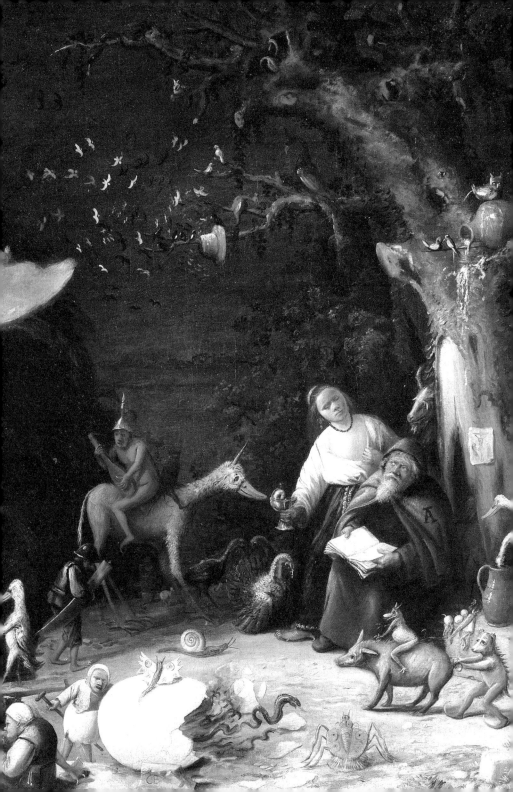

multiply, they were to embrace chastity. Clement's instructions were part of a larger programme of asceticism: the faithful were to refrain from drinking and eating too much and exchange their fine clothes for sackcloth.

***

The early Church's most-influential champion of the idea that desire was wicked was Augustine of Hippo, a fourth-century bishop from modern-day Algeria. He was, ironically, no stranger to the carnal delights of imperial Roman society. Before he converted to Christianity in 392, he was a brilliant young orator on the make in Italy, where pampered Roman elites dedicated themselves to the pursuit of luxury and sensuality. "I ran wild in the shadowy jungle of erotic adventures," he recalled in his autobiography, *Confessions*. One such adventure lasted 13 years. He evidently cared about his lover, for when he ended the relationship, due to his engagement to a wealthy ten-year-old girl, he was deeply upset. Augustine was not so heartbroken, however, that he couldn't bring himself to acquire a new concubine during his long engagement. "A chain of habit, its links silently formed around his will in the course of 13 years of unproblematic enjoyment of sexual companionship, now held him fast," writes historian Peter Brown. Augustine famously implored, "Lord, give me chastity and continence – but not now."

Even after he converted to Christianity, Augustine found it terribly difficult to cast aside this chain of habit. Though he had renounced sex, his dreams still pulsed with forbidden fantasies which concluded with nocturnal emissions. This perturbed him: though a man could move his arms and feet around at will, when it came to his sexual organs, they would "not obey the direction of the will, but lust has to be waited for to set these members in motion, as if it had legal right over them".

Augustine saw in his body's insubordination a metaphor for original sin. The body disobeyed the self just as Adam and Eve disobeyed God, not by having sex, as the ascetics argued – Augustine believed that God had intended them to have sex – but by desiring each other. As Augustine saw it, sex in paradise was a rather dry affair. The mind governed the genitals as it did the rest of the body, and intercourse brought with it none of the delirious pleasures of orgasm. But when Adam and Eve defied God by letting their bodies be ruled by lust instead of the will, God came up with a clever punishment: the flesh would never again obey the mind as it had in

Saint Augustine Praying *(1636)*
by Jusepe de Ribera

Eden. Augustine wrote:

> When the first man transgressed the law of God, he began to have
> another law in his members which was repugnant to the law of his
> mind, and he felt the evil of his own disobedience when he experi-
> enced in the disobedience of his flesh a most righteous retribution
> recoiling on himself.

That desire was sinful was of course a familiar idea in the early Church. But for most Christians, it was one temptation of many, a temptation that could be conquered through the free exercise of the will. Augustine believed otherwise. In a cruel twist, Adam and Eve infected their descendants at the moment of conception with original sin, which was passed on from one generation to the next. This meant that no matter how virtuously humans behaved, they could never wash away the stain of desire, which served as an eternal reminder of their ancestors' catastrophic mistake. Salvation could be achieved only through the grace of God.

Desire weighed heavily on Augustine, yet he did not condemn all sex. He believed that God smiled down upon sexually active married couples as long as they had intercourse for the right reason – procreation – and in the right way: passionlessly. Couples had to do their best not to let lust lead them into sin, as it had Adam and Eve.

Augustine's conception of desire greatly magnified its importance to the understanding of the self. In classical antiquity, desire was just one arena in which a citizen could demonstrate his self-control, assert his social status and prove his moral worth to fellow citizens. Accordingly, sex in the Roman world was governed by the "laws of the forum". Augustine, however, thought it fell under the jurisdiction of a higher power: the "laws of heaven". Desire didn't just threaten to compromise one's social standing – it endangered the soul. Any time lust flickered within the body, it was an echo of original sin: the individual would have to decide whether to succumb to temptation, like Adam and Eve, or resist it – a struggle in the eyes of Augustine that defined what it meant to be human.

***

The Church Fathers believed that Eve was to blame for original sin. It was she, "the devil's gateway", who was deceived by the serpent and convinced Adam to join her in disobedience. This interpretation of Genesis justified the belief that women, daughters of Eve, were not only evil instruments of the Devil but inferior to men and subject to them. Woman's punishment was subordination in marriage and the desperate dangers of childbirth.

Despite Christianity's overwhelmingly negative view of Eve's descendants, many women converted with zeal. There were practical advantages for female believers. Pagan culture regarded women as chattel, but those who gave their lives to Christianity could attain spiritual authority. In the second and third centuries, when Romans persecuted Christians, devout women who refused to recant their faith were marched into arenas and brutally executed or torn apart by wild beasts. Confronted with these dazzling displays of heroism, the Church Fathers had to concede that in martyrdom, women were the equals of men.

In later centuries, when Christianity was legalised and the faithful could no longer prove their piety in the Roman arena, many women resolved to follow the example of Thecla, who by now was legendary for her feats of asceticism. The life of the ascetic afforded these "new Theclas" a measure of independence. Virginity delivered women from marriage and motherhood and, according to the Church Fathers, would help them to regain the status they lost in paradise. Wealthy, aristocratic women travelled to the Holy Land, founded and ran monasteries, and studied the scriptures. Some joined an order of deaconesses, who helped bishops teach women the basic tenets of the faith. In eastern Christendom, deaconesses were even ordained.

But by the end of the fourth century, the Church Fathers were determined to bring women to heel. They agreed that women could not be priests or public teachers and that they had to accept a diminished role within the Church. Though religious life still held attractions for women, what formal power they had was subsumed under the authority of a male hierarchy. Increasingly, if they wished to live a life of celibacy, they had to become nuns and join convents.

***

In the fourth century, Christianity strode triumphantly from the shadows of the realm into its throne room. Emperor Constantine converted in 312 and by the end of the century Christianity was the official religion of the empire. Thecla had formally banished Venus – yet many citizens still worshipped at her altar. Only five to ten percent of those within the Roman Empire actually practised Christianity. Sometimes even the clergy behaved more like pagans than Christians. By the fourth century, the Church was urging priests to renounce sex but many got married anyway and, if ditties sung at a pagan Roman fertility party in 495 are to be believed, frequently cheated on their wives. Over a century later, the governor of Syracuse appointed the local bishop to the post of Imperial Inspector of Brothels. The pope was appalled by the news – though not perhaps shocked.

It would take a millennium for Christianity to fully lodge in the souls of Europeans. Yet in the last years of the empire there were signs that it had found a perch. Eroticism was viewed with growing suspicion. Spiritual advisors now asked young men whether they were still virgins – a question which, three centuries earlier, would have been asked only of young women. Attitudes to homoeroticism hardened. In the fourth century, a bust of Antinous, the beloved of Hadrian, a second-century Roman emperor, was re-carved so that he resembled an imperial lady.

Behaviour that violated the Church's sexual code of conduct was gradually treated with greater severity. Shaped by Christian thought, fourth-century imperial decrees banned any sexual activity between spouses that did not involve the insertion of the penis into the vagina. In the fifth century, it became illegal for men as well as women to commit adultery. And in the sixth-century, Justinian, the emperor of the eastern Roman Empire, imposed the death penalty for same-sex sex ("because of such crimes there are famines, earthquakes and pestilences," he declared) and banned divorce by consent in what amounted to the harshest moral law code the empire had ever seen. The Codex Justinianus enshrined Christianity as the law of the land. Thecla was there to stay.

CHAPTER THREE

DOING UNTO OTHERS: THE MIDDLE AGES

There is one evil, an evil above all other evils, that I am aware is always with me, that grievously and piteously lacerates and afflicts my soul…This evil is sexual desire, carnal delight, the storm of lust that has smashed and battered my unhappy soul, drained it of all strength and left it weak and empty.

So anguished is this passage, you would be forgiven for thinking it's an excerpt from Augustine's *Confessions*. It was actually written hundreds of years later by St Anselm, the 11th-century Archbishop of Canterbury. Much had changed since Augustine's day. The Roman Empire had crumbled, and over its ruins a new elite – the pope, with his cardinals, bishops and priests – had steadily built an institution capable of instructing, punishing and purifying souls. The approach of the millennium, and with it the conviction that Judgement Day was nigh, had concentrated minds on the conquest of sin, but when the apocalypse failed to materialise, Europeans turned their focus from life after death to life before it. Sleepy towns were jolted awake by the cries of tradesmen and the clink-clink of merchants' moneybags; by students at newly opened universities making merry and troubadours who wandered from castle to castle, entertaining nobles and monarchs with songs of forbidden love. Looming over them all by the 12th and 13th centuries were Europe's new Gothic cathedrals, their towering spires potent symbols of the Catholic Church's vast power. Now the West's dominant religious institution, it had also become a significant force in politics and society.

Even as Augustine's Rome faded from memory, his doctrine of original sin tightened its grip on Christendom. As St. Anselm's tortured confession makes all too clear, desire was regarded with horror. The most devout Christians proved their spiritual vigour by embracing chastity permanently, along with a life of prayer and penance. Yet medieval theologians, recognising that most people were not able or willing to abstain forever, agreed with the Church Fathers that, while desire was wicked, sex could be justified if a married couple wished to have children. Though these Christians did not share in the heroism of virgins, they could still be considered chaste as long as they observed the Church's definition of virtuous sex.

This concession was reflected in a new and enduring Christian system of categorising social groups which supplanted the old Roman hierarchy. As Caesarius, sixth-century Bishop of Arles, declared in a formula that would be repeated throughout the Middle Ages: "Indeed there are three professions in the holy Catholic Church: virgins, widows and the married. Virgins produce a hundredfold reward, widows sixtyfold, the married indeed thirtyfold." Classifying people according to how much sex had touched their bodies was a way of indicating their relationship to the Church. "Virgins" and "widows" stood for men and women who had taken holy orders and vows of chastity – primarily monks and nuns, medieval successors to ascetics like St Anthony – while the "married" symbolised laymen and women who only had Church-sanctioned sex. The Church refused to officially acknowledge anyone who was simultaneously unmarried and sexually active. In its idealised vision of Christian society, everyone was either valiantly virginal or chastely married.

∗∗∗

Some people never married – in northern Europe as many as 15 percent

– but matrimony was the fate of most. The medieval Church sought to control their sex lives by elaborating an unwieldy list of rules couples were commanded to observe. Christians were to be monogamous and sexually faithful to their spouses; they were also to refrain from divorce and exhibit restraint during sex, the timing of which was restricted. Couples had to abstain during certain holy periods of the Church calendar such as Wednesdays, Fridays and Sundays and most major saints' days, plus all of Lent and Advent. Sex was also prohibited when the wife was menstruating, pregnant or nursing a child. There were so many constraints on the timing of intercourse that those who observed them would have been at liberty to tangle in the bedroom just 50 days a year.

The rules did not end there. There were regulations on the time of day (night only), the proper attire (almost fully clothed), the position (missionary, with the man on top) and location. Couples were to stop having sex in churches. That this needed to be said may surprise some readers but consider the average medieval house: smokey, muddy and heaving with people and animals, it was so small that most couples did not have their own bedrooms. Churches were safe, dry and empty for much of the day – "the medieval equivalent of the back seat of the car," as historian Ruth Mazo Karras puts it. Clerics, however, didn't want the upholstery to be soiled, so joyriders were warned off, and instructed not to darken the church's doorstep again until they had washed.

Not content to dictate when, where and how its flock was to have sex, the Church also wanted to make sure people were doing it for the right reasons. Having sex for the pleasure of it was a mortal sin, as devotees of St Jerome regularly reminded their flocks when they parroted his line: "A man who is too passionately in love with his wife is an adulterer." Married couples were to lie together calmly and decorously, their bodies set in motion only by God's command to go forth and multiply.

That the Church felt the need to formally set down these regulations suggests that many medieval people did not have the sexual comportment of good Christians. But even those believers who did want to follow the rules might have been confused, for they were riven with contradiction. Even as the Church condemned pleasure, it implicitly condoned conjugal lust by telling married couples that they were not allowed to refuse each other sex. A chaste marriage was still the ideal – St Alexis was much ballyhooed for abandoning his wife's bed on their wedding night – but only if both partners were game. The Church did not want one spouse's abstinence to drive her help-meet to adultery; it also did not want to empower medieval Lysistratas to rebel against their husbands by denying them sex. So it decreed that couples were to fulfil their "marriage debt" to each other. If a wife failed to render her husband his due (or vice versa), she was responsible for any sin he might commit by, say, masturbating or embracing another woman. In its efforts to shore up the institution of marriage and the rights of husbands over their wives' bodies, the medieval Church came to a conclusion that would have appalled St Jerome: servicing a spouse's desires was more virtuous than being chaste.

**

Rules were pointless unless the Church could enforce them. The early Middle Ages witnessed the emergence of confession, which allowed priests to probe the souls of their parishioners and punish any sins they detected by meting out penance. Determining which sins were more sinful than others was a bit tricky so in the seventh century the Church started issuing handbooks to confessors which ranked transgressions in order of magnitude and prescribed the penalty for each. The largest single category of offence related to sex. These sins are described in such prurient detail that one historian contends that the intended audience for these books – celibate clergymen – must have been "fascinated by sex".

The least serious of these sins of the flesh, according to one influential 11th-century penitential, were male masturbation and fornication with an unmarried woman. The lenience with which these infractions were punished (ten days on bread and water and no sex) reveals how tolerant society was of the youthful indiscretions of unmarried men. Far more consequential were abortion and the use of contraception, which earned ten years' penance: this meant abstaining from sex and eating nothing but bread and water on the Wednesday, Friday and Saturday of each week and the annual fasts of Christmas, Easter and Pentecost. The most egregious sins – incest, sodomy and bestiality – warranted the greatest penalty: 15 years.

These sex acts horrified the late-medieval Church because they seemed like perversions of God's will. According to St Thomas Aquinas, a 13th-century Italian theologian, God designed humans to be rational. Any sexual act that is irrational – meaning, basically, any act that is not procreative – contradicts human nature and is therefore "unnatural" (Aquinas also used the term "sodomy" to refer to sex acts that could not lead to conception). Which sexual acts were identified as "unnatural" varied: one theologian argued that vaginal intercourse with the woman on top counted because she couldn't get pregnant in that position. Typically the category encompassed bestiality, anal and oral sex, any sexual act between two members of the same sex and, increasingly in the later Middle Ages, masturbation. So much did the Church abhor unnatural sex that Gratian, the pre-eminent canon lawyer of the age, insisted that incest was preferable to something like masturbation because it was "natural".

***

The Church's policies governing the groin were the harshest western Europe had ever known. And by the 12th century, it was better able to enforce its rules thanks to the establishment of its own permanent courts and the Inquisition, which enabled bishops to discipline their flocks quickly. Yet there is evidence to suggest that the Church's efforts to bend the laity to its will were not a resounding success. For one thing, people may not have gone to confession more than once a year. For another, clerics themselves observed that fornication was rampant. The old idea that young, unmarried men should be able to sow their wild oats was so entrenched – even the penitentials let male fornicators off lightly – that, by 1287, the Church felt the need to declare such a view heretical. Spoiler alert: it made little difference.

The Church's anxiety is revealing. For all its power, it could not stamp out alternative attitudes to sex. Though many believers no doubt internalised Christian morality, common people cared more about fertility than snuffing out their desires and tried to ensure conception with pagan spells and rituals. Comic folk tales about the consequences of insatiable lust had peasants in stitches, while romantic tales exalting adulterous love, sung by bards and troubadours, entertained aristocrats. Meanwhile, translations of Latin, Greek and Arabic texts on medicine and science put surgeons, artisans and merchants in touch with the intellectual worlds of other cultures.

No matter whether rustic or royal, godly or godless, everyone understood sex as a reproductive act. In an age without reliable methods of birth control, biology fundamentally shaped attitudes to sex. Doctors did not encourage abstinence. Medical experts thought that regular intercourse was essential to health. This theory derived from the ancient view of the body as a kind of human cauldron bubbling with four fluids – blood, phlegm, yellow bile and black bile – the balance of which shaped one's personality and health. It was believed that males maintained the correct admixture in their bodies by sweating, bleeding or emitting semen during the night. Men were advised to help things along by ejaculating periodically but always in moderation – over-indulgence could injure the health as much as abstinence.

Though the female body was, according to the ancient theory discussed in Chapter One, very similar to the male body, it wasn't as hot and didn't produce as much sweat. With fewer outlets at their disposal to regulate the balance of humours, as those liquids were known, women relied particularly on ejaculation (the female body was thought to produce semen), which is why doctors maintained that abstinence was particularly harmful for women. To relieve the pain caused by the build-up of ejaculate, some medical manuals actually encouraged midwives to manipulate the genitals of virgins and widows until they climaxed.

Some medical authorities also believed that if the uterus was not regularly purged through sex or menstruation, it would start to emit lethal fumes or even float up through the body towards the head, causing the woman to faint or die. There were a variety of methods for treating this condition, including wrestling the womb back to its original position, but it could be avoided entirely by regular intercourse.

Doctors not only discouraged abstinence; some even urged husbands to consider their wives' pleasure. The ancient theory of reproduction, which held that conception relied on mutual orgasm, was still influential. Accordingly, some manuals recommended foreplay, and instructed husbands to kiss their wives, fondle their breasts and massage their pudendum. The Middle Ages was a grim time to be a woman – the daughters of Eve were universally regarded as temptresses and naturally subject to men – but at least this theory of conception encouraged husbands to attend to their wives' sexual satisfaction.

It was not, however, a theory that was universally accepted (other experts believed that conception relied on male orgasm only) and some of its implications were unfortunate if not downright nasty. Women who wished to avoid conception would have tried to avoid climaxing, while any woman who was impregnated after being raped was legally considered to have consented to intercourse. She couldn't have fallen pregnant, the thinking went, without also enjoying the experience.

**

Like their ancient Greek and Roman counterparts, medieval women were regarded as sexually insatiable. In Chaucer's *Canterbury Tales*, the Wife of Bath is matter-of-fact about her erotic temperament:

Venus gave me desire and lecherousness
And Mars my hardihood, or so I guess.
I ever followed natural inclination
Under the power of my constellation
And was unable to deny, in truth,
My Chamber of Venus to a likely youth.

To modern readers, the Wife is empowered: she enjoys sex and will fandango with whomever she pleases. But the idea of an independent woman was meant to be ludicrous and a little frightening. The Wife is ruled not by reason, as men are, but by the wild desires of her body. Would men ever be able to satisfy her? In one *fabliau*, a comic French tale, a husband grumbles to his wife, "Lady, you have a greedy mouth in you that demands to be fed too often. It has tired my poor old war-house out." Male authors of popular literature often fretted that voracious female desires would make a mockery of their sexual prowess.

Female passion could subvert the sexual hierarchy – but only momentarily. If anything, transgressive female behaviour reminded society of the natural order of things: that sex was, ultimately, something that men did to women, as Karras argues, not something that men and women did together. No matter how active the Wife's desire, she played the passive role in sex. She might initiate a sexual relationship, she might even assume a dominant position during intercourse, but it was her husband who penetrated her, not the other way around. And he was permitted to do so against her will. When a woman married a man, she gave him the right to have sex with her at will. Rape did not exist in the marriage bed.

**

Anyone who eavesdropped on the men gathered in the bath-houses and barber shops that sprang up with the urban revival of the 12th and 13th centuries would have heard them eagerly plotting their next "hunt" for "Ganymedes" – slang for cruising for attractive young men. The first stirrings of the Renaissance were kindling interest in the classical world – hence the reference to Ganymede, Zeus's cup-bearer – but this literary enthusiasm did not translate into toleration of physical expressions of same-sex love. Sodomy was a carnal sin "so abominable", Pope Gregory XI shuddered, "that I dare not mention it." (At the time, "sodomy" technically referred to "unnatural" sex acts but colloquially it referred to sex between males.) But despite the threat of being consigned to the seventh circle of Hell, as Dante predicted, large numbers of men persisted in committing this "unspeakable" act. In 1102, St Anselm, Archbishop of Canterbury, wrote that hitherto "the sin has been so public that hardly anyone has blushed for it." Male brothels were said to operate in Chartres, Orléans, Sens and Paris. Florence, Dante's hometown, was so notorious for its sodomites that in Germany such men were known as *Florenzer*.

Florence deserved its reputation. Late-medieval European societies encouraged men to become attached to each other. Close friendships were formed in schools, guilds and monasteries; apprentices and journeymen worked together, caroused together and shared beds at night; young hopefuls at court or in the Church curried favour from their male superiors. But Florence took it to another level. At night gangs of men prowled the streets in pursuit of beautiful young Ganymedes, who had long hair and wore tight, colourful stockings. Once a man had captured his prey, the pair would decamp to a quiet alley or an empty garden. If a man couldn't pick anyone up on the street, he might swing by one of the taverns frequented by youths eager to service older men. Or maybe he would strike lucky at work. Men and boys employed at butchers' shops and groceries on the Ponte Vecchio were known to have sex with each other. So common was sodomy, across all levels of Florentine society, that in the late 15th century the majority of local men would be officially incriminated for it at least once in their lifetimes, as historian Michael Rocke has shown.

Sodomy was prevalent in Renaissance Florence not because women were unavailable – the city teemed with prostitutes and concubines – but

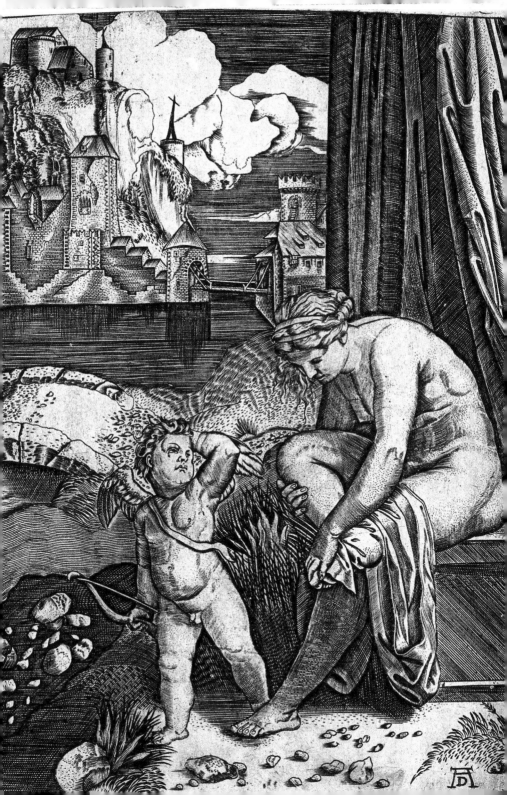

because the local masculine culture, based as it was on hierarchical bonds between older and younger men, quietly permitted it to flourish. Usually short-lived, male relationships were characterised by a disparity in age, much as they were in ancient Greece. Older, more established men pursued poorer youths on whom they lavished gifts and personal favours. For every year that they were together, Leonardo da Vinci bought Salai, a beautiful boy with darling curls, 24 pairs of shoes and even gave his sister a dowry. (Such relationships could be so lucrative, fathers sometimes encouraged their sons' trysts.) If Leonardo wished to avoid being deeply transgressive, he would have penetrated Salai during sex, for the active role was the part played by manly men, while the passive role was feminine and humiliating. However, as the submissive role was normally limited to late adolescence, it was merely a temporary diversion on a boy's journey to manhood.

Though late-medieval Florentine society did not condone sodomy, it was punished sporadically. That changed in the early 15th century. In the 1420s plague was ravaging the city. Bernardino of Siena, a charismatic preacher, began to deliver sermons that blamed the epidemic on sodomy. Not long after, Florence created the Office of the Night, the sole purpose of which was to root out and punish sodomy. This was in keeping with a wave of persecution that swept through Europe during the 13th and 15th centuries. Before, the Church had treated sodomy with relative leniency; the punishment was comparable to that for adultery. But by the late-12th century, theologians had reframed sodomy as both a violation of nature and the most evil of sins. In 1215 the Church decreed that sodomites would be excommunicated. Not long after, the rulers of England and France mandated death by burning for sodomites. But it was in Florence that the most systematic persecution of any premodern city took place – not that it stopped da Vinci.

***

Even as Florence cracked down on Ganymedes, it was profiting from prostitution. In 1403 the city's Office of Decency established a municipal brothel and licensed prostitutes and pimps to work in it. Florence wasn't the first city to regulate prostitution. Venice opened a brothel in 1360; over the next hundred years, a slew of towns in Italy, France and England followed suit. Far from turning a blind eye, the Church got in on the act and leased property to brothel keepers, making a tidy sum in the process.

Ganymede, a mythical Greek figure whose beauty so captivated Zeus, the king of the gods, that he turned himself into an eagle and abducted him

Towards the end of the Middle Ages in the 15th century, the papacy was pocketing 28,000 ducats a year from this sideline. Privately, the pope must have agreed with Venice's Grand Council when it described prostitution as "absolutely indispensable to the world".

On what grounds? According to the Church, the only legitimate outlet for sex was marriage. But cities were full of young men who were deferring marriage until their late 20s in order to establish their careers. In the meantime, these lads were drinking in taverns, brawling, raping respectable women, cavorting with men and frequenting prostitutes. Medieval society idealised men who were dominant and aggressive but these young men were out of control. Religious and secular authorities who had long attempted to put a stop to prostitution began to think of it as a necessary evil. Surely it was better for a young man to have sex with a prostitute, who was already polluted, than to seduce a virgin or commit sodomy? Aquinas wrote, "The prostitute in society is like the sewer in a palace. If you take away the sewer, the whole palace will be contaminated." The authorities concluded that, as the sewer needed to remain in place, they might as well make some money out of it. Municipal brothels sprang up all over Europe.

***

Clerics were not permitted to use brothels. From the 12th century, the Church made priests take vows of celibacy; the spiritual authority of the clergy was, after all, supposed to derive from their chastity. Yet rumours of priests seducing or even raping penitents during confession abounded, and thousands of clergymen across Europe were prosecuted for keeping concubines. Nuns slipped up too. In the 13th and 14th centuries, 33 Venetian convents faced criminal charges for illegal sexual activity. That these men and women were disciplined by the Church is ironic considering the sexual proclivities of their pontiffs. Prostitutes openly serviced clients at the Vatican. For a party he once held at the papal palace, Pope Alexander VI hired 50 whores to dance with the guests. An observer recalled:

At first they wore their dresses, then they stripped themselves completely naked. The meal over, the lighted candles, which were on the table, were set on the floor, and chestnuts were scattered for the naked courtesans to pick up, crawling about on their hands and knees between the candlesticks.

Familiar with bawdy stories mocking clerical lechery, most people shrugged off the sexual pastimes of the clergy as minor sins. Not Martin Luther – a German monk – who was horrified by the corruption and dissipation of the Church. Sex was at the heart of his critique. Clerical debauchery was proof that permanent chastity was all but impossible, Luther argued. Desire was so strong a force that resisting it was fruitless: "To say it crudely but honestly, if it doesn't go into a woman, it goes into your shirt," he said. The best Christian life, even for clerics, was one that channelled lust into wives. In 1525, Luther renounced his vows and married a former nun.

Luther's rejection of clerical celibacy was part of a broader attack on the Church. He wanted believers to establish their own relationships with God, unmediated by priests. By branding the pope the "Whore of Babylon" and rejecting Church doctrines like the authority of the papacy and the importance of tradition, Luther undermined the clergy's status as

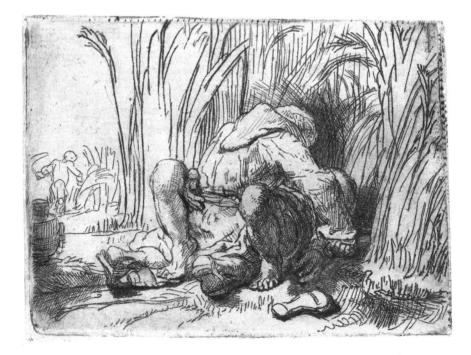

Vow of celibacy? What vow of celibacy?
The Monk in the Cornfield *(1646) by Rembrandt*

intercessors with God. His ideas sparked widespread revolt. Many secular rulers, eager to curtail the economic and political power of the papacy in their territories, broke with the Catholic Church and established their own churches, which came to be called "protestant". By the 1530s, much of northern Europe, including England and Scandinavia, had followed suit. It quickly became clear however that the division in Christendom would not stop with Luther. As a host of different groups – Zwinglians and Calvinists among them – advanced different interpretations of the Bible, the unity of Christendom shattered. Conflict between Protestants and Catholics would pitch Europe into over a century of war.

The Reformation gave rise to a new social hierarchy of the faithful. The Catholic Church evaluated people according to how much sex had touched their bodies, and accorded supposedly pure, celibate monks, nuns and priests the highest status. But Luther denounced celibacy and encouraged everyone to express their sexual desires in marriage. His celebration of the passion which flows "naturally" between men and women led him to condemn the unnatural behaviour of sodomites. This idea was not new of course – the Catholic Church abhorred sodomy. But it didn't exactly approve of spouses who had ordinary sex with each other either, and because it believed that everyone was infected with original sin, the Church anticipated, and forgave, sinners. By contrast, Protestants were perfectionists. They were convinced they could snuff out all ungodly desires. This conviction impelled them to more-rigidly divide humans into male and female, whose lust for each other was natural, and sodomites, whose desire for each other was not.

This perfectionism created a regime of sexual discipline that was far more rigorous than that which had preceded it. Protestant authorities did not tolerate extramarital sex. Brothels were closed. Adultery became a capital offence in Scotland, Puritan England and parts of Protestant Germany. Sex before marriage was harshly punished, though men had an easier time of it than women. There was widespread support for these measures. Popular hostility towards those who violated sexual norms grew and as the number of illegitimate births declined in early-modern England, so did – we can infer – the number of people who had premarital sex. The religious fervour of the age resulted in a widespread sexual puritanism, one that would eventually be attacked from an unlikely quarter.

CHAPTER FOUR

PHILOSOPHY BETWEEN THE SHEETS: THE ENLIGHTENMENT

Through the keyhole, Thérèse spies an extraordinary sight. Her dear friend, Eradice, is kneeling on a prayer stool, her skirts lifted up to her waist to expose her buttocks. Standing behind her is Father Dirrag, her confessor. Eradice had invited Thérèse to secretly observe her "spiritual exercises" with the priest in order to prove how, with his help, her soul is able to slip the bonds of flesh and steal into God's embrace. But Thérèse is uneasy about the hungry look on Dirrag's face. "Only by forgetting the body can we find unity with God," he intones, as he starts to flagellate her posterior. As Eradice prays, thinking she is entering into communion with the Lord, the priest enters her from behind with his swollen member, which he pretends is a holy relic. Innocent Eradice is becoming one with her confessor, not God.

Thérèse is overcome with horror, as much by her own arousal as by the priest's deception. When as a young girl she was caught masturbating, her confessor taught her that her nub of pleasure was the very apple that seduced Adam and caused the Fall of man. But not long after the episode with Father Dirrag, Thérèse leaves the convent, where she was a student, and encounters the philosophy of the Enlightenment. She learns that God is a human invention, that truth can be discovered only by reason, and that the aim of life is the pursuit of happiness in this world not the next. After a liaison with a female prostitute, she concludes that sensations so delightful can't be wicked. She strikes up a sexual relationship with a count; they pleasure each other and philosophise together – happiness is attained.

When this metaphysical cumming-of-age tale was published in France in 1748, *Thérèse Philosophe* was an underground hit. The novel, thought to have been written by Jean-Baptiste d'Argens, an aristocratic philosopher, belonged to a wildly popular genre of "bad books" as the police called them. This genre traced its origins to early 16th-century Italy, when the first sexually explicit prints, poems and pamphlets, made with the intention of arousing those who bought them, were produced.

These bad books weren't pornography, per se. *Thérèse Philosophe* didn't just titillate; it attacked the Catholic Church as well as the sexual mores of the era. In early-modern Europe (in other words between 1500 and 1800), the pornographic novel was "most often a vehicle for using the shock of sex to criticise religious and political authorities", as historian Lynne Hunt points out. Society did not distinguish between pornography, heresy, political subversion and intellectual radicalism (pornography would not be recognised as a category unto itself until the early 19th century). Indeed, the French government of the *ancien régime* lumped together all works that threatened the Church, the state or conventional morality and labelled them "philosophical books", no matter "whether they were politically motivated scandal sheets, metaphysical treatises, anticlerical satires or pornographic stories", Hunt writes.

The term was apt. Many authors of pornographic tales were themselves philosophers or intellectuals. Benjamin Franklin penned erotic poems. Voltaire, Mirabeau and John Wilkes, a British champion of free speech, wrote saucy stories. Diderot was locked up in 1749 not just for declaring his atheism but for writing erotica – his contemporaries even suspected he was the author of *Thérèse Philosophe*. There is little evidence for such a claim, but the connection is understandable. Diderot was determined to liberate Eros from the Church's clutches. Like Thérèse, he believed that sexual appetite was natural and that its repression was pointless; that the goal of life was to be happy – in this world – and that sexual passion would

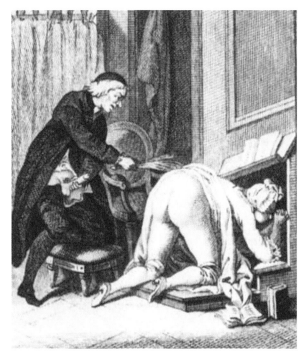

Eradice and her confessor enter into communion with each other. From the hit 18th-century novel, Thérèse Philosophe

contribute to that effort. As Diderot wrote, "There is a bit of testicle at the bottom of our most sublime feelings and our purest tenderness." With the growth of cities and literacy and the spread of print culture, philosophers of the Enlightenment could communicate their ideas through plays, pamphlets and novels. Fictional characters like Thérèse could be summoned to show readers who might not otherwise crack open a work of philosophy why a spot of testicle-tickling, far from condemning them to hellfire, could introduce them to heavenly delights.

***

That Diderot could thumb his nose so brazenly at over a millennium of Christian teaching marked a seismic rupture in the intellectual landscape, one that would throw the moral puritanism of the age off balance. The conditions for this rift were long in the making. In some parts of Europe, the power of Christianity as a political institution and intellectual force

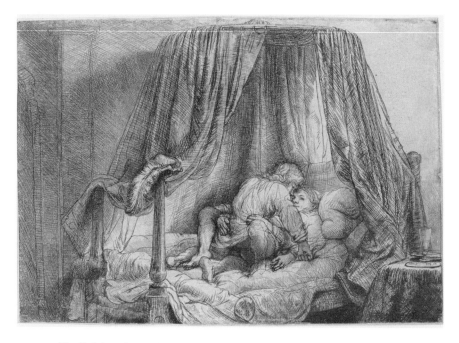

The Bed *(1646) by Rembrandt. A rare contemporary depiction of a couple having sex*

was on the wane. The Reformation had shattered the unity of the Catholic Church. In the ensuing centuries, increasingly powerful secular rulers gradually denied their local Churches the right to discipline the morality of the public. In 17th-century Calvinist Europe, secular courts began to wrest jurisdiction over sexual matters from Church courts. In 1689, England granted freedom of worship to all Protestant sects, fatally undermining the ability of ecclesiastical courts to police public morals.

As Protestant European states began to undercut their local Churches' ability to discipline sexual behaviour, the scientific revolution of the 16th and 17th centuries challenged Christian theology. By demonstrating that the universe operated according to mathematical laws, Galileo and Newton seemed to strip God of His mystery. Philosophers familiar with the new science fastened on to a bold idea: God was a divine watchmaker who had designed nature as a kind of mechanism, set it in motion and then departed. Nature was no longer a realm that could be made intelligible only through divine revelation; it could be understood rationally.

This scientific revolution sparked intellectual debates that would eventually loosen the era's stays, as historian Faramerz Dabhoiwala has shown. In the second half of the 17th century, English thinkers began to argue for religious freedom; their success would lay the foundations for sexual toleration. At the time, the idea that ordinary people should follow their consciences without the assistance of scripture, teachers or laws was considered ludicrous, especially because sinful behaviour risked not just an individual's salvation but that of the entire community. However, thanks to the new science, God was viewed more as a benevolent figure removed from the daily affairs of humans. The centuries-old idea that divine retribution would wipe out entire cities began to seem antiquated. In 1689 John Locke, an English philosopher, argued that, in fact, an individual's spiritual beliefs did not jeopardise the well-being of society, and therefore those beliefs were not the business of government. Conscience was a personal matter. This didn't in itself advance the cause of sexual freedom but it would lead to a sharp distinction between public and private life, creating the conceptual space necessary to argue that what one did in one's bedroom was not the business of the state.

Such a notion was buttressed by Locke's argument that punishing people for their innermost beliefs was pointless because it never changed their minds (as centuries of religious wars showed). This fatally undermined the long-standing belief that penalising those guilty of sexual crimes would reform their behaviour. If people's consciences could not be compelled, the punishment of sexual transgression lost much of its justification. Within a few decades, the predominant view in England held that true penitence could not be forced by laws. It could perhaps be encouraged by education and charity, but ultimately had to come from within. Magistrates were to focus on crime, not sin.

But if the state wasn't going to tell you how to behave, how, exactly, was one's conscience to determine right from wrong? The spread of religious pluralism in England, the rise of deism in France, and the cries of freedom in the American colonies had made the presumption that one should blindly obey the Church seem old-fashioned. The modern view held that one ought to ascertain moral truths logically and that nature – interpreted by one's senses and experiences – should be the measure of morality. Mainstream Enlightenment thinkers tried to reconcile Christianity with natural law, but radicals rejected Christianity, claiming that its moral precepts – among them the requirement to be chaste – weren't God-given at all but merely priestly inventions. God's real laws, which were simple and rational, could be found only in nature. And anyone who looked to the fields and farmyards would see an abundance of care-free rutting, for in nature sexual liberty was the rule. As David Hume, a Scottish philosopher, wrote, "confinement of the [sexual] appetite is not natural".

Others went further. The Enlightenment elevated the pursuit of happiness as the most important goal in life. Sexual satisfaction was clearly one way of attaining it – perhaps the only way. Pleasure was "the principle of life and energy" that animates love, commerce and society itself, Diderot wrote. "I desire therefore I am." Two other 18th-century French thinkers were even more radical. Julien Offay de La Mettrie and the Marquis de Sade dismissed not just religion but all metaphysics. As materialists, they believed that knowledge of the world could only be gained through the senses. Life, they said, is composed solely of matter which is predisposed to motion; they considered sexual desire, which impels matter to move toward other matter, to be a kind of energy. Desire and all sexual proclivities, no matter how unorthodox, were natural because they sprang from the body. "Have we the power to remake ourselves?" asked de Sade. "Can we become other than what we are?" Of course, the answer was no, so the very idea of restraining sexual behaviour was illogical. For de Sade, "pleasure defined morality", as historian Eric Berkowitz writes.

Such ideas were dangerous. La Mettrie was exiled to Berlin; de Sade was imprisoned. But materialism would live on in the pages of one of the most widely read "bad books" of the century: *Thérèse Philosophe*. Its probable author, Jean-Baptiste d'Argens, a radical deist philosopher notorious for his many mistresses, "used materialist philosophy to challenge the authority of the Church with the authority of the body", writes Anna Clark. Having discarded Catholicism as a bastion of hypocrites and sophists, Thérèse becomes a devotee of reason and materialism. All life can be reduced to matter in motion, and as she discovers, having her own matter put in motion is deeply pleasurable.

***

The cause of sexual libertarianism was championed by the libertine, an individual who married free-thinking with free-living, to borrow Robert Darnton's formulation. Libertinism first flourished in England during the

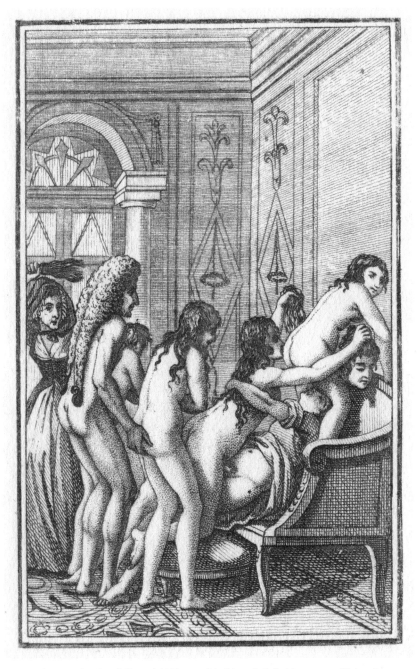

An engraving from Juliette *(1797), one of the Marquis de Sade's pornographic novels*

reign of Charles II (1660-1685), whose court – still reeling from the severity of life under Oliver Cromwell's Puritan regime – eagerly embraced these new ideas. The Earl of Rochester scorned religion as no more than "the jugglings of priests" and believed lust "was to be indulged as the gratification of our natural appetites." The entire court soon became "absorbed in an endless game of sexual musical chairs", as Lawrence Stone puts it.

Libertinism gradually spread beyond the palace gates. At first the English public regarded the notion that unconstrained lust enhanced masculinity, rather than diminished it, with disgust. The orthodox view held that womanisers lacked self-control and would be disciplined by God. But Charles's court made sexual promiscuity fashionable. Men of the English upper crust were soon expected to have many mistresses – Lord Keeper North was sternly advised to find one lest he "lose all his interest at court".

By 1713, *The Guardian* was tut-tutting that the cult of seduction had become so modish among the haut monde that for a man to aspire to chastity had "become ridiculous". Rakes availed themselves of condoms and dildos, which first became available in London in the 1660s, and from the early 18th century, joined exclusive societies for sexual experimentation. Renowned for its bacchanalian orgies, the Hell-Fire Club, established in 1719 for the purpose of ridiculing conventional morality and religion, was later rumoured to include among its members Horace Walpole and the Prince of Wales. The market soon began to respond to this movement. By the early 18th century, those who wished could purchase pornographic prints, which were widely produced and distributed, and of course, novels. Published in 1748 (the same year as *Thérèse Philosophe*), *Fanny Hill* is still to this day probably the single most-read pornographic novel of all time.

***

By the mid-18th century, there had emerged in Europe and the American colonies a doctrine of sexual liberty grounded in a new understanding of natural law and personal liberty. What one did with one's own body was a private matter, as long as it was "natural" – "unnatural" sex was now defined as sodomy and masturbation – and did less harm than good. Articulated at a time when the pursuit of happiness was becoming a political ideal, this doctrine opened up the possibility that individual pleasure could be the goal of sexual congress rather than procreation or duty to a spouse.

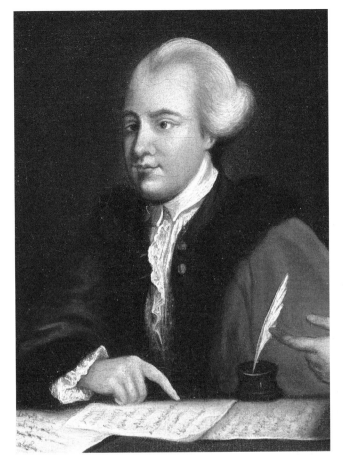

The credo of the libertine was summed up in 1763 by John Wilkes, a
British politician: "Life can little more supply / than just a few good
fucks, and then we die"

However, this belief system was by no means intellectually dominant.
Though it was increasingly accepted that all men were naturally predisposed to fornication, most men and women continued to do their best
to live up to traditional ideals of chastity. And the principle of personal
liberty applied only to certain people. "In every civilised society", observed
Adam Smith in 1776, there existed two different moral codes: a "loose"
one for the fashionable and a "strict" one for commoners.

Smith was not entirely right. It is true that it was primarily gentlemen
and noblemen who invoked philosophy to justify libertinism, while sexual

propriety was often held up as a distinguishing feature of the emerging middle class. But the forces shaping the sex lives of working people were shifting. From the middle of the 18th century, the number of European women who gave birth out of wedlock skyrocketed. Before, a young buck who impregnated his sweetheart would probably have submitted to pressure from his community to marry her. But in the newly industrialised economies of the late 1700s, a man could easily abandon his girl and his village and find work in the booming cities. Many did. Once they had escaped the traditional expectations placed on them by their communities, a large culture of urban, mobile men – labourers, sailors and tradesmen – disported themselves in pubs and brothels. These men weren't libertines, but there was liberty to be found in the anonymity of cities where they could explore sexuality outside of marriage. By the end of the century, people from a broad cross-section of society "began to consider the 'sins of the flesh' as harmless and natural," writes historian Stephen Garton.

***

For all the ink spilled in defence of sexual liberty, almost everyone agreed that some sexual acts were still "unnatural". Samuel Stevens certainly did. One evening in 1725, he paid a visit to Margaret Clap's house in Holborn, a tatty neighbourhood in London. What he saw there appalled him:

> I found between 40 and 50 men making love to one another, as they called it. Sometimes they would sit in one another's laps, kissing in a lewd manner and using their hands indecently. Then they would get up, dance and make curtsies, and mimic the voices of women.

Stevens had walked in on a gathering of sodomites, or "mollies" as they were popularly known. Margaret Clap's house was one of several in London that catered to men who wished to have sex with other men. There were similar such establishments in 18th-century Paris and Dutch Harlem, cities where subcultures of men with such proclivities were emerging.

These groups set themselves apart from the dominant sexual culture with rituals and coded language. In London's molly houses, "When any member entered into their society, he was christened by a female name, and had a quarter of a pint of Geneva thrown in his face; one was called Orange Deb, another Nell Guin, and a third Flying Horse Moll." Mollies spoke in distinctive ways – "calling one another 'my dear' and...assuming effeminate voices and airs" – and aped female fashions. "Some were dressed like milkmaids, others like shepherdesses..." Before couples retired to the back-rooms, they would announce they were repairing to the chapel to be married. After "consummating" the union they would divulge details of their "wedding night" to friends, who would not have been overly concerned about who assumed the passive or active role. Unlike men with similar sexual inclinations in 15th-century Florence or ancient Greece and Rome, mollies freely switched between roles.

Belonging to these subcultures was dangerous. In the early 18th century, sodomites were ruthlessly persecuted in the Netherlands and England. From 1699 to 1726, the Society for the Reformation of Manners, a crusading English organisation to which Stevens probably belonged, periodically instigated raids on molly houses which led to mass arrests, trials and executions attended by huge, gleeful mobs.

This wave of persecution in England was unlike any that had come before it. Though sodomy had been punishable by death since the 13th century, individuals had been prosecuted only sporadically. Now entire groups of people were being executed. It's not that English society was now more offended by men who had sex with each other. On the contrary: the sodomite had been so reviled in Renaissance England that natural disasters – catastrophes attributable only to God's rage – were blamed on him. Yet despite the fear and revulsion the sodomite inspired, the "unmentionable sin" of which he was emblematic often went unmentioned. Sodomy was easily ignored. Casual same-sex liaisons happened frequently – at schools and universities, in households and theatres – but sodomites were difficult to identify. Nobody publicly announced he was one and most of these men also had sex with women. Rumours that Francis Bacon slept with his male servants, or that the mid-16th century headmaster of Eton dallied with a former student, were more difficult to disregard, but the image of the sodomite was so extreme that society was often reluctant to expose such people. So same-sex behaviour was effectively tolerated in early-modern England – as long as it was discreet.

That changed with the molly. He was an individual whose appearance, behaviour and way of life all singled him out as a sodomite. Being a molly meant one was a particular kind of person, with a particular identity: that of a man who had sex exclusively with men. But precisely because mollies were identifiable, they were more difficult for society to ignore and easier for the authorities to target.

***

For men, sexual liberty clearly had its limits. What about women: were there any real-life Thérèse Philosophes? The radical Enlightenment created the intellectual conditions necessary for them. A few who thought seriously about sexual liberty acknowledged that chastity was as unnatural

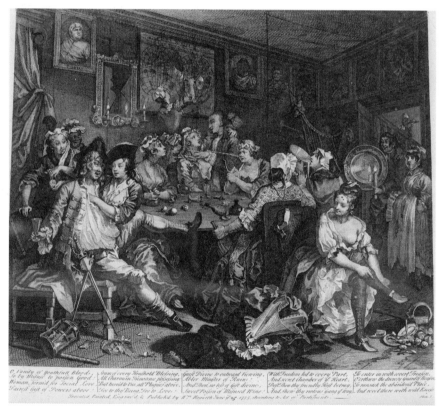

The third scene of William Hogarth's series, A Rake's Progress *(1735), in which Tom Rakewell disports himself with prostitutes in a Covent Garden tavern*

for women as it was for men: by 1740 Hume thought this "so obvious", it did not need explaining. Some women paid heed. In revolutionary Paris, where intellectual circles were still digesting Diderot's assertion that sex should be enjoyed for the sake of it, Mary Wollstonecraft, an English philosopher, fell madly in love with an American entrepreneur. They scorned marriage and surrendered to those "sensations that are almost too sacred to be alluded to," as she wrote to him. Several years later, Wollstonecraft herself wrote a novel, *Maria, or The Wrongs of Woman*, defending the right of women to sexual freedom.

Wollstonecraft, however, was unusual. Very few writers publicly endorsed the right of women to have sex with whom they pleased. Most defended the traditional view, that women should be chaste, for the same patriarchal reasons that have echoed through the centuries. Unfaithful wives would foist bastards on their husbands, muddying the family bloodline and threatening the patrimony of legitimate children. Because "all property in the world depends" upon the chastity of women, as Dr Johnson wrote, wifely infidelity could not be considered a harmless or private matter. And single women like Wollstonecraft faced consequences easily avoided by men. Without reliable forms of birth control, female libertines could become pregnant.

In fact, even as 18th-century men revelled in their newfound sexual freedom, English women were increasingly being portrayed as sexually passive, as Dabhoiwala shows. This was a remarkable development. Since the dawn of western civilisation women had been regarded as the more lecherous of the two sexes. Lust, of course, bedevilled all humans, but women, regarded as less rational, less virtuous and less disciplined than men, were believed to be much more susceptible to it, as the story of Adam and Eve proved. So when in 1621 Robert Burton railed: "of woman's unnatural, insatiable lust, what country, what village doth not complain?" he was merely expressing the conventional wisdom of the age. But had Burton posed the question 200 years later, he would have complained about the moral corruption of his own sex. For the 1700s turned conventional wisdom on its head: it made women out to be delicate, sexually passive creatures forever at risk of being seduced by men, who were now seen as naturally lecherous. By 1800 this view of female sexuality was so entrenched that Eve herself was no longer seen as Satan's help-meet but as the original seduced woman. The libertine, wrote the author of *Advice to Unmarried Women* (1791), was to be avoided "as the serpent that beguiled the first of your sex".

Men were presumed to be naturally rapacious because they were behaving, well, rapaciously. From the late 17th century, restraints on male libidos loosened. As we have seen, intellectual arguments in favour of personal liberty began to erode those championing male chastity. In practice, male sexual discipline was undermined by the fatal weakening of Church courts and, with the rapid growth of cities, the decline of local communities' ability to regulate morals as they had done for centuries. With the formalisation of English justice in the early 18th century and the skyrocketing expense of litigation, it became more onerous for moral reformers like Stevens to bring charges against people like Mother Clap. And as the Lockean view that government should butt out of the private lives of citizens gained traction, adulterers and fornicators gradually stopped being treated like public criminals. "By 1750 most forms of consensual sex outside marriage had drifted beyond the reach of law," Dabhoiwala writes (sodomy was a notable exception). Some of the most important curbs on predatory male behaviour had started to disappear.

A new kind of writer sounded the alarm. By the late 17th century, British women's voices had begun to be heard on the stage and page. Before, men had monopolised every medium in which the proper roles of men and women were formulated and entrenched, from drama, poetry and journalism to sermons, theology and philosophy. But in the late 17th century, women began to pick up their quills. Their plays, poems, novels, pamphlets and works of philosophy portrayed women as the virtuous victims of rakish men who were fickle if not downright cruel. As Mary Astell, a philosopher, said in 1700, "'tis no great matter to them if women, who were born to be their slaves, be now and then ruined for their entertainment."

Earlier models of masculinity had focused on relations between men, largely ignoring women. But by the 18th century, English and American women, having been inferior in virtue and self-control, were increasingly seen as the moral superiors of their male counterparts (an idea the French had advanced a century earlier). According to this new ideal of politeness, unruly men would be tamed and civilised by the serene influence of women. There was no "better school for manners, than the company of virtuous women," as Hume said.

For all the talk about women bringing men to heel, however, the primary consequence of this new ideal of civility was to restrict *female* behaviour.

If women were going to be celebrated for their purity, they had to live up to the ideal. Doing so became increasingly difficult as charming, insistent men, their libidos no longer kept in check by societal norms, queued up to "ruin" them for sport. In a letter to a suitor written in 1710, Lady Mary Wortley Montagu summed up the different experiences of courtship for men and women: "'Tis play to you, but 'tis death to us."

The idea that men were naturally licentious and women chaste began to be scientifically defended. Even as 17th- and 18th-century sex manuals popularised the ancient idea that female orgasm was necessary for conception, physicians and natural philosophers began to disprove it. They argued that conception occurred independently of any "tell-tale shivers", as Thomas Laqueur puts it, on the part of the woman.

The demotion of the female orgasm was part of a more radical late 18th-century reinterpretation of the female body in relation to the male. By 1800 scientific advances, among them the discovery of the clitoris, had chipped away at the classical theory that women had the same basic anatomical make-up as men. Women were no longer seen as lesser men; their bodies were fundamentally distinct. Doctors now said they could identify "the essential features that belong to her, that serve to distinguish her, that make her what she is" – a sex apart from men. By 1800, society justified female subordination by invoking biology and psychology rather than scripture or the classical humoural body. As the English moralist John Brown wrote in 1765, it was from women's "delicacy of body" and "delicate timidity of mind" that "the great female virtue of chastity ariseth on its strongest and most impregnable foundations".

Not everyone accepted such a view. Speaking through Maria, the heroine of her novel, Wollstonecraft argued that the notion that women are fragile and frigid was degrading:

> When novelists and moralists praise as a virtue a woman's coldness of constitution and want of passion, I am disgusted. We cannot, without depraving our minds, endeavour to please a lover or husband, but in proportion as he pleases us. Men, more effectually to enslave us, may inculcate this partial morality, but let us not blush for nature without a cause!

Nobody who knew Wollstonecraft could accuse her of delicacy. Having made the case that women, being capable of rational thought, should be treated as the equals of men, she proceeded to behave as a sexually liberated bachelor might, by conducting several love affairs. In her embrace of sexual freedom, Wollstonecraft embodied Thérèse Philosophe, but unlike her, Wollstonecraft suffered the consequences of her radicalism. Several months after bearing her American lover a child, he abandoned her. She raised her daughter by herself, eking out a living from her writing. Wollstone-craft's life and work served to undermine the now-dominant conception of women as "passionless", which explains why, when she died in 1797 from complications during childbirth (her daughter, Mary, would survive and go on to write *Frankenstein*), conservatives laid waste to her reputation, attacking her as a deranged feminist whore. The backlash against the idea that liberty should reign in the bedroom had begun.

Mary Wollstonecraft, a British Thérèse Philosophe

CHAPTER FIVE

RESPECTABLE SEX: THE VICTORIAN AGE

The year was 1798. The Enlightenment idea that society was improving and, in theory, perfectible, was encountering resistance. In revolutionary France, the first shoots of democracy had been hacked down by Robespierre and then rooted up by the Directory. Across the Channel, deep in the English countryside, a clergyman named Thomas Malthus had just finished writing *An Essay on the Principle of Population*, which painted a bleak picture of the future. Like the Enlightenment philosophers, Malthus believed sexual desire was an irrepressible natural force, but he regarded this force with fear, for he believed that population growth would inevitably outstrip the food supply, leading to famine and death. He was right that the population was swelling. Between 1700 and 1835, Europe's population doubled, with birth rates soaring in particular from 1750. People were having more sex, both in and out of wedlock; a third of all brides were pregnant in 18th-century England and the US. For many in the West, Malthus's warning was a rude awakening from the Enlightenment's dream of desire as a positive force. Fearful that rampant population growth would cause surges in crime and lead to revolt, governments began to realise that desire needed to be carefully managed.

It was out of this context that an ideology of domesticity developed in early-19th-century England. The libertinism of the upper classes, and the sexual libertarianism of radicals like Wollstonecraft, had always caused the pious to purse their lips in disapproval. As a wave of religious enthusiasm swept through the country from the late 18th century, their reproach gained force. When revolution erupted across the Channel, many argued that it was the inevitable consequence of the *ancien régime's* licentiousness. As a correspondent of the *Public Ledger* wrote in 1816:

> That the French Revolution, with all its constant horrors, was preceded by a total revolution of decency and morality, the virtuous qualities of a mind being sapped and undefined by the baneful exhibition of pictures, representing vice in the most alluring and varied forms, to a depraved mind, is a truth that unfortunately will not admit of doubt.

It was clear to evangelicals that the libidinousness of aristos led inexorably to the disintegration of society. Such a fate, they argued, could be staved off in Britain as long as the foundations for a new, stable society were laid on the bedrock of the family rather than the loose morals of the libertine. Evangelical intellectuals like William Wilberforce and Hannah More began to describe the family as a Christian haven in a storm-tossed world, and urged those who would listen to embrace piety and sexual decorum, even in marriage. Though Protestantism had always celebrated desire between husband and wife, evangelicals and radical Protestants, in both England and America, began to emphasize sexual restraint, even abstinence.

As the 19th century progressed, this moral framework was adopted by the English bourgeoisie, which was increasingly politically and economically powerful and keen to distinguish itself from the morally lax upper and lower orders ("fit only for sleep or sensual indulgence", as one moralist sighed). This moral code found expression in an etiquette of "respectability" that drew clear lines between decent, hard-working, morally upright members of society and everyone else. A tell-tale sign of the former was their prudery, a quality personified by Mrs Grundy. A fictional character who became a symbol of Victorian censoriousness, she looked on approvingly as matrons took down the cheeky 18th-century prints from their drawing-room walls, Wedgwood covered up the nude figures on his pottery, Bowdler scrubbed the filth out of Shakespeare and the Bible, and genteel men and women bowdlerised their own conversation, referring to chicken bosom, for instance, rather than chicken breast. Mrs Grundy had affixed a fig leaf over Victorian sexuality. The respectable were not supposed to talk about sex, or even think about it.

Married couples were the exception to this rule. From the late 18th century, the upper classes had idealised romance between husband and wife; in the early 1800s, the bourgeoisie began to follow suit, casting marriage as an institution in which both partners would fall in love with each other and find ultimate happiness. This rhetoric encouraged Victorian spouses to think of sex not just as an obligatory prelude to procreation but as a means of kindling intimacy between each other. In the Victorian era, new rules prevented the consummation of such intense feelings until after the couple had married. In the 18th century, it was acceptable for couples to start having sex once they were betrothed, but new marriage laws passed in the early 19th century had the effect of making betrothals less binding, sharply distinguishing the married from the unmarried, and licit sex from illicit sex. The conjugal bed was now the only acceptable venue for sex.

If marriage was now the gateway to respectability, home was its setting. As news of political and social unrest in England and Europe dominated headlines in the 1830s and 1840s, home was idealised by many moralists, writers and poets as a sanctuary from strife – "the shelter not only from all injury, but from all terror, doubt and division," as John Ruskin, an art critic, put it. That the "vestal temple" could loom so large in the Victorian imagination was thanks, in part, to industrialisation, which relocated workers out of the house, where they had plied their trades for centuries, into the factory and office.

As work and home were prised apart, they became potent symbols of another divide, between men and women. The 18th-century notion that the sexes were biologically, psychologically, intellectually and morally distinct had become definitive by the 19th century. As a result, gender became one of most important social categories of the Victorian age. As historian Angus McLaren observes, "Western culture had always stressed male and female differences but in the 1800s gender became privileged, often eclipsing one's rank, status, profession, race or religion as the key determinant of personality." Governed by reason, men were the natural occupants of the world of work – the public sphere – while women, ruled by sentiment, belonged in the home, the private sphere.

This rhetoric prescribed strict rules of behaviour for the middle class: women were to be quiet, virtuous and meek, guardians of the home and hearth, while men, channelling the new ideal of the thrifty, cautious businessman, were supposed to exercise restraint. Expected to fortify themselves against the stresses and dangers of the wider world, men were not to let emotions or weakness – marks of femininity – find the chinks in the armour of their manhood. From the 1860s, a new cult of masculinity in England ensured that men no longer dared cry or embrace in public, for fear of being ridiculed as womanly.

The 18th-century idea that women were naturally chaste and men lascivious was confirmed by 19th-century medicine. Popular medical treatises and works of sexology, the emerging science of sex, defined male sexuality as direct, forceful and instrumental, while female sexuality was seen as responsive, expressive and shaped by female emotion. Some medical advice writers continued to stress that husbands must take care to please their wives sexually, but many others believed that women's sexual pleasure was unimportant and their libido mild, if it existed at all. Havelock Ellis, a British sexologist, noted that this effort to deny female sexuality as "a vile aspersion" was particular to Italy, Germany, the United States and Britain. One of the most famous exponents of this idea was William Acton, an English doctor, who in 1865 wrote that "the majority of women (happily for them) are not very much troubled by sexual feelings of any kind."

Many middle-class women accepted this view. It allowed them to claim spiritual authority over men, and gave them a reason to refuse the sexual advances of their husbands. But this view of female sexuality was by no means universal. In her rejection of Acton's theory, Elizabeth Blackwell, a pioneering woman doctor, characterised female sexuality as an "immense spiritual force of attraction" and an "impulse towards maternity". Missing from Blackwell's theory, and indeed all 19th-century thought, is the notion that women had sexualities independently of men's, as historian Jeffrey Weeks observes. If women were believed to experience sexual feelings, they were seen as finding their fulfilment in motherhood. Instead of undermining this view, the century's scientific breakthroughs – the discov-

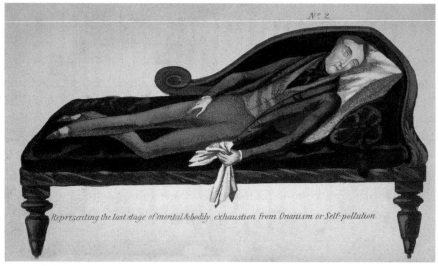

Representing the last stage of mental & bodily exhaustion from Onanism or Self-pollution

An illustration from 1845 depicting the harmful effects of masturbation or "Self-pollution"

ery of the role of ovulation in the menstrual cycle, for instance – were used to confirm traditional ideas about women's sexuality.

∗∗∗

Though evangelists of respectability enjoined both men and women to behave with sexual propriety, the ideology of separate spheres held women to a much higher standard than men. Many husbands struggled valiantly with temptation as they strove to live up to the ideal of married life, but it was women who suffered if they succumbed. In France, unfaithful wives could be prosecuted by the state under the Napoleonic Code and imprisoned for up to two years. By contrast, husbands could not be penalised for straying and could only be divorced if they brought their mistresses home.

Adulterous wives were punished by society as well as by the law. The new ideal of the passionless woman created its mirror opposite: the fallen woman who failed to resist men's advances. In the past, the woman who repented her sins could be welcomed back into the community, just as a contrite man would be. But her Victorian counterpart was believed to occupy a higher moral plane than men; her fall from such heights was so great it ruined her for life. "Even as woman is supremely virtuous," wrote an American novelist, "when once fallen [she becomes] the vilest of her sex."

Though English society idealised men who practised self-restraint, it was much more forgiving of promiscuity in men than women. Libertine attitudes persisted. In 1848, Charles Dickens told a foreign visitor that "[male] incontinence is so much the rule in England that if his own son were particularly chaste, he should be alarmed on his account, as if he could not be in good health." Nobody could accuse Dickens of sickliness. Like many middle- and upper-class men, he kept a mistress. Others turned to prostitutes. As professional men delayed marriage later, the prospect of respectable sex becoming ever more remote, the incentive to avail themselves of commercial sex grew. Respectable society frowned, but sleeping with a prostitute was not illegal and such behaviour was widely regarded as both the inevitable consequence of male needs and a way of safeguarding wives from seduction. It even found tacit approval from the government. In 1871, a Royal Commission commented that solicitation was to be regarded as no more than "an irregular indulgence of a natural impulse".

Evidence that gentility was not universally embraced could be difficult to ignore on certain streets in Paris and London. Driving through the Bois de Bologne in well-appointed carriages, wealthy, elite courtesans known as the *grandes horizontales* caught the eye of passing gentlemen, while their English sisters paraded down Regent Street, Oxford Street and "the chief temple of frippery and frivolity", the Burlington Arcade. So well dressed were English prostitutes that passers-by often could not tell them apart from respectable women. As the *Saturday Review* fretted in 1862, it was difficult "to make out the true character of a vessel from the colours under which she sails". But lady shoppers gliding down the Burlington Arcade had to pretend not to notice as leering men mistook them for prostitutes. Respectable women were not supposed to acknowledge when desire overstepped the bounds of propriety.

For some women, this was difficult to accept. During the 1850s Josephine Butler, a feminist who lived in Oxford, learned that a don was rumoured to have seduced a "very young girl" who bore him a child. She confided in a man whom she believed to have integrity that she hoped the don would be brought to a "sense of his crime". He replied that a "pure woman...should be absolutely ignorant of a certain class of evils in the world". For women, Butler wrote, "silence was thought to be the greatest duty of all on such subjects." As historian Hera Cook observes, "The dominant sexual culture in mid-Victorian Britain was shaped by the acceptance of purchased sexual relief for men and respectable women were forbidden to discuss it."

Stung by this hypocrisy, some women refused to shut up. From the 1860s, English middle- and upper-middle-class women who were angry about the double standard sought to establish a single standard of morality – that of the chaste woman. They set their sights on that vice most intimately associated with the public sphere and the world of men: prostitution. In doing so, they tapped into a mounting concern among the English public, and that of other western European countries: that the "social evil" of prostitution was growing and venereal disease spreading.

National governments grew alarmed. In the last decades of the 19th century Germany and Italy, seeking to manage the spread of venereal disease, imitated France by instructing the police to register and regulate prostitutes. Though the British had resisted intervening in the private lives of citizens since the early 18th century, the prevalence of the disease among its soldiers – up to 30 percent in the imperial army – worried the top brass. Officials responded by demanding the inspection of the women soldiers slept with. The Contagious Diseases Acts (CDA) required that prostitutes register with the authorities and submit to compulsory medical examinations, first in Hong Kong in 1857, then in English and Irish garrison and port towns by 1864.

Many women, Butler among them, decried state regulation for implicitly condoning male lechery. Across Europe, female activists began to agitate for repeal. During the 1870s and '80s, Butler led a mass movement in England for the revocation of the CDA. She presided over a large coalition of feminists, social-purity activists, and working-class men angry that the Acts "endanger the liberty and virtue of their wives and daughters while those of the men of the upper classes are safe". While working men framed the issue in terms of the class struggle, social-purity activists invoked the traditional Christian association between sexuality and sin, and Butler spoke for feminists when she argued that the problem posed by prostitution was not female immorality but male lust. The way these women spoke about sex was powerfully negative, and contributed to a growing perception of sex as dirty, diseased and sinful.

Over the last two decades of the century, and the first decade of the next, female activists grew in influence. A string of causes and scandals sustained an alliance composed of feminists like Butler and social-purity reformers as they sought to lift the country out of the gutter. The drive to improve standards of morality was nothing new, of course, but the efforts of early-19th century evangelicals had been checked by the fear of revolution. No such fear haunted later campaigners, who were galvanised by what was seen as a decline in moral standards during the 1850s and 1860s, and who acquired a "new articulateness about sexual morality", according to Lesley Hall, thanks in part to the entry into the public sphere of those who had previously been ostracised, including feminists and nonconformists.

Emboldened by their success with the CDA, which was repealed in 1886, social-purity campaigners continued to attack the double standard, distributing thousands of pamphlets urging men not to visit prostitutes and – with even greater urgency – not to masturbate. Activists idealised continence so much, some even suggested that married couples should restrain their sexual appetites. "In the sight of God," Edith Ward proclaimed, "immoderate indulgence of the passions is as offensive between" married people as between unmarried people.

***

Social-purity campaigners were so successful that they changed the tone of public life. The irony is that even as women activists muscled their way into the public sphere, their negative slant on sexuality contributed to growing female ignorance about sexuality and reproduction, as Hera Cook argues. Respectable Victorian women had not always been innocent of matters sexual. Early- to mid-century accounts indicate that women like Effie Gray, whom Ruskin married in 1848, had intense physical desires which they felt able to express. When Ruskin refused to consummate their marriage – for religious reasons he wished to delay the moment by five years – Gray secured an annulment.

But in the last third of the century, many middle-class women, and some men, knew far less about sex, and were less able to enjoy it. When he got married in 1897, the architect Edwin Lutyens lacked sexual experience, and his wife Emily later told her daughter that the honeymoon was "a nightmare of physical pain and mental disappointment". During inter-

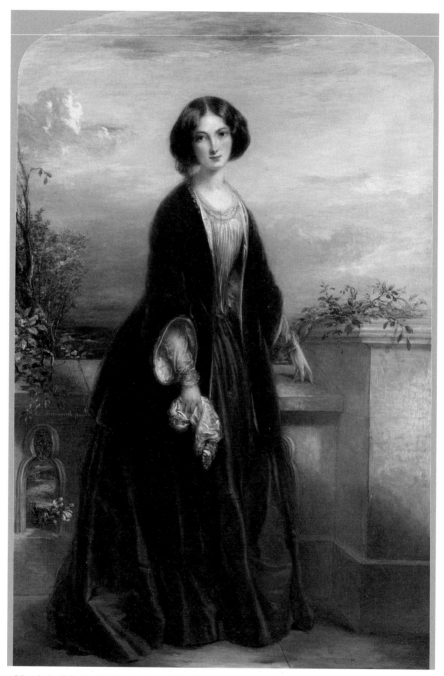

Married to John Ruskin for five years, Effie Gray eventually secured an annulment because he refused to consummate the union

course, Edwin evidently proceeded rapidly and with little awareness of Emily's feelings, making the experience "increasingly disagreeable" to her, one she came to find "disgusting". The culture did not permit Emily to make sexual demands of Edwin, and because premarital sexual petting had long since been stigmatised, she was unlikely to have known how she might have been sexually and emotionally satisfied. It is also possible that neither Emily nor Edwin understood how to express affection. By the mid-19th century, middle-class families were no longer physically demonstrative. Spouses may have expressed fondness for each other behind closed doors, but the chances that children would observe their parents' affection, and learn how to communicate such emotions themselves, diminished. The effects of this were amplified down the generations.

The Lutyenses were victims of a shift in the sexual culture of the middle class, one that ushered in an era of sexual restraint – even within marriage – that would last well into the 20th century. This new era coincided with a sharp decline in fertility. After soaring from 1750, the West's birth rate plummeted dramatically in the following century, first in France and the US, then in England after 1870. At the beginning of the 19th century the average English woman had eight children; by 1925, that number had dropped to two. Mechanical methods of contraception were not widely available in the beginning of the century, and there was widespread resistance to its use later on, so Cook argues that middle-class English men and women were spacing births by having less penetrative sex.

There were many voices in the late 19th century urging couples to limit the number of children they had. Neo-Malthusians recommended delaying marriage, minimising the childbearing years of the wife. The first feminists, seeking to spare women unwanted pregnancies, also called for sexual moderation. But considering how little authority wives had over their husbands, Weeks thinks it likely that changing perceptions of the appropriate family size were more significant in reducing fertility than "domestic feminism". Like their wives, husbands wished to maintain a certain standard of living. During the economically straightened circumstances of the late 19th century, middle-class couples responded to the rising cost of education, for instance, by limiting their fertility.

By the end of the century, the birth rate of the working class was declining, suggesting a shift in working-class sexual mores similar to that which had first taken place among the middle class a couple decades earlier.

Fearful that industrialisation was destroying family life by encouraging women to seek employment in factories, Victorian evangelists of middle-class respectability sought to improve the morals of the working class. Yet this reduction in fertility had less to do with the imposition of middle-class values on the working class and more to do with the latter's cultivation of its own, distinct ideology of respectability. For the hard-working, God-fearing proletariat, this code of behaviour demanded that he provide for his wife and children so that they would not need to work. It followed that when money was tight – as it often was in the difficult economy of the late 19th century – couples limited the number of children they had.

Historians broadly agree that they spaced births by practising *coitus interruptus* as well as abstinence. (Abortion was a last resort for many women, particularly in factory districts, where knowledge of abortifacient techniques was widespread.) The ideology of respectability that emerged among the working class in the last decades of the 19th century was marked by a deep sexual conservatism and an equally profound ignorance of the mechanics of sex.

✳✳✳

The respectable working-class family man would have been horrified by what he saw in London's glittering shopping districts. Rubbing shoulders with the local prostitutes were men who went cruising for men. As London's population expanded, a greater degree of anonymity became possible for the increasing numbers of men joining a homosexual subculture that had embedded itself in city life, as it had in Paris, Berlin and New York (that "city of orgies, walks and joys", according to Walt Whitman). A guidebook to London's pleasures published around 1855 noted that "Margeries" and "pooffs" could be identified by their "effeminate air and fashionable dress" and could be found in theatres, coffee houses and London's shopping Meccas, strengthening the association of homosexual behaviour with fashion, effeminacy – and transactional relationships. "Will the reader credit it", the guidebook tittered, "that these monsters actually walk the streets the same as whores, looking out for a chance!"

As Margeries became more visible in London, the police stepped up their response. During the 18th century, policing of the capital had been patchy and disorganised; the persistence with which men frequented cruis-

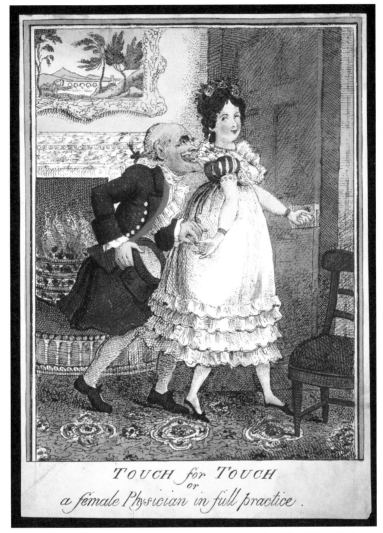

*TOUCH for TOUCH
or
a female Physician in full practice.*

*In this print (1811), Thomas Rowlandson puns on the word "touch", which at the time
meant both to have sexual contact with and successfully get money out of somebody*

ing areas suggests that periodic waves of prosecution, like those endured by
the mollies of Mother Clap's house, did not totally deter men from return-
ing. But in 1829 with the establishment of the Metropolitan Police Force,
policing became more rigorous. Bobbies were given increased powers to
monitor the behaviour of suspected Margeries: they began to monitor
streets at night, watch men cruising in alleyways, and haul those accused

of indecent behaviour into magistrates courts alongside drunks and prostitutes. The police did their best to prosecute such men quietly, in order to
avoid public scandal and limit public knowledge of such crimes.

Even as the police tried to keep such men out of the papers, mid- to
late-Victorian social-purity campaigners began to concentrate minds on
homosexuality. As we have seen, reformers were preoccupied with male
lust, which they believed was to blame for both prostitution and homosexual activity. They worried that male dissipation in all its forms threatened
the sanctity of the marriage bond, the family – even imperial security.
To the social-purity advocate, the strength of the family guaranteed the
strength of the empire; because homosexuality threatened the family, it
threatened the country too. "Rome fell; other nations have fallen; and if
England falls it will be this sin, and her unbelief in God, that will have
been her ruin," one purist wrote.

It was in this climate that legislation concerning homosexuality was
refined. For centuries, homosexual activity had been criminalised under
an act passed in 1533 by Henry VIII punishing sodomy "with mankind or beast". In the second half of the 19th century, the law began
to pinpoint homosexual acts. In 1885 the Labouchere Amendment to
the Criminal Law Amendment Act punished any "male person who, in
public or private" committed any "acts of gross indecency with another
male person". This expanded the scope of the law by specifically criminalising sexual relations between men, no matter where they took place.
By the late 19th century the domestic sphere was thought of as a zone
governed by the family rather than the state. As Matt Cook points out,
the Amendment reminded the British that such acts were illegal, no
matter whether they happened in public or private.

While the Labouchere Amendment specifically targeted male homosexual acts, the Vagrancy Law Amendment Act (1898) criminalised
homosexual identities by letting the police arrest men they thought might
be homosexual. When, one evening in 1912, plainclothes policemen
observed an actor entering public toilets in Piccadilly Circus – a known
cruising spot – they apprehended him. The police reported that, though
he didn't make contact with anyone, "he smiled in the faces of gentlemen,
pursed his lips and wiggled his body" and wore make-up. No one had complained about him but he was dragged into court anyway and sentenced
to ten weeks' hard labour, not for having illegal sex but for looking and

behaving like a man who might have such sex.

The late-19th-century laws were formally less repressive than the 1533 buggery act – they replaced the death penalty with jail sentences – but they were for this reason more likely to lead to convictions. And by sending out "powerful messages about expectations of private conduct and public behaviour", as Cook puts it, they created a repressive environment. Men who expressed homosexual inclinations were threatened with exposure, potential prosecution and public disgrace. A flurry of sex scandals helped to define the boundaries between acceptable and unacceptable behaviour and assisted the new laws in their effort to suppress homosexuality.

The most famous scandal of the century concerned the Irish playwright, Oscar Wilde. In the late 1880s and early 1890s, Wilde and other intellectuals began to articulate their desires more openly than homosexuals had dared before, writing homoerotic poetry for privately published journals and wearing green carnations, which symbolised their sexuality. When Wilde published a novel, *The Picture of Dorian Gray*, in which a character champions a "new Hedonism, that was to recreate life, and to save it from that harsh, uncomely puritanism", his enemies claimed that it celebrated homosexual desire. The novel would be used in 1895 to convict him of "gross indecency" under the Labouchere Amendment. He was sentenced to two years' hard labour, a punishment which ruined his health and destroyed his career. Ironically, however, his trials publicised homosexuality, creating a public image of the male homosexual and a sense of identity. According to Havelock Ellis, the trials appeared "to have generally contributed to give definiteness and self-consciousness to the manifestations of homosexuality, and to have aroused inverts to take up a definite stand." Two years later, Magnus Hirschfeld, a German reformer, created the first organised movement dedicated to the emancipation of homosexual men. As homosexuality became more prominent, a small group of scientists – Hirschfeld and Ellis among them – would begin to study the sexualities of "deviants" like Wilde in a new discipline called sexology.

CHAPTER SIX

THE DOCTOR IN THE BEDROOM: SEXOLOGY

In the early 1930s, a young man sought the help of a Parisian psychiatrist named Pierre Vachet. This man, whom Vachet called "Pierrette",
was highly unusual: he said he had the soul of a woman. Pierrette had
delighted in wearing women's clothes ever since he was a boy but, with
time, he realised he wanted to be a woman rather than play the part of
one. He struggled with this desire for several years but eventually decided
to renounce his life as a man. He wore dresses and make-up in public; he
shopped, cooked and cleaned. Pierrette's relief was immediate. His depression lifted and he finally felt able to be himself.

There was just one thing missing: Pierrette longed to be able to per-
form sexually as a woman. In his account of the case, Vachet observed
that the kind of sex change Pierrette wanted had already been performed.
But Vachet believed that surgery was insufficient for people like Pierrette.
Because the nervous system caused transsexuality, he wrote, it should be
treated with psychotherapy.

Vachet's account of Pierrette marks how far this history has travelled since the dawn of the Christian era. To the Catholic Church, sexual deviancy was sinful; to secular society, it was unnatural; and to the state, it was criminal. But by the early 20th century, some doctors began to reject these ways of thinking about deviance. They argued instead that sexual perversions were symptoms of psychological disorders.

These doctors worked in a new field of biomedical science called sexology. Richard von Krafft-Ebing, an Austro-German psychiatrist and one of the discipline's founding fathers, articulated the view of his colleagues when he wrote in 1886, "Few people ever fully appreciate the powerful influence that sexuality exercises over feeling, thought and conduct... The importance of the subject demands that it should be examined scientifically." Along with a handful of doctors and psychiatrists based in Germany, Austria, France and Great Britain, Krafft-Ebing believed that by defining, categorising and labelling the various forms of sexual desire, he not only could, but must, produce an objective science of sexuality. For if deviants were sick, there was a chance they could be cured.

***

For centuries, the priest had been the expert and arbiter on sexual desire. But the Enlightenment had popularised the view that nature would only give up her secrets to those who could methodically observe, measure and label her. The 18th century had engendered the faith that those who correctly applied this scientific method to the human body would discover how it functioned. Physicians began to investigate sexuality. Biomedical researchers studied reproduction and the workings of the sexual organs, discovering in the 1830s the processes of ovulation, menstruation and fertilisation. In the second half of the 19th century, medicine was professionalised and accorded greater scientific and social status; new specialities like public hygiene and psychiatry rapidly expanded. "More and more, physicians, acting as mediators between science and the vexing problems of everyday life, succeeded in convincing the public of the indispensability of their expertise," notes historian Harry Oosterhuis. Though Christian Churches would continue to wield influence over sexual matters, by the end of the 19th century, the doctor had slowly but surely edged the priest wout of his role as the ultimate authority on sex.

Lili Elbe, born Einar Wegener, was one of the first transsexuals to receive a sex change, in Berlin in 1930. This watercolour was painted by her wife in 1928

Sexual deviance was becoming increasingly difficult to ignore in certain parts of the Western city. Growing numbers of men seeking anonymous sexual encounters with other men met in parks, theatres, bathhouses, pools, public toilets and railway stations. The public nature of these liaisons, along with the growth in the number of streetwalkers, led to confrontations with moral reformers who considered such behaviour an affront to public decency and demanded stricter law enforcement. The establishment of professional police forces in western Europe and the United States from the early- to mid-19th century brought more criminals before the courts than ever before.

As a result, magistrates were increasingly called upon to adjudicate sex crimes. As they confronted behaviour that was more difficult to comprehend than rape or sodomy – from exhibitionism to the sexual compulsions of serial killers – European magistrates often summoned doctors to help them make sense of such acts. As Angus McLaren writes, "The prosecution of such crimes required that the boundaries separating permitted and forbidden, 'normal' and 'abnormal', sexual practices be rigidly drawn."

To establish those boundaries, doctors first had to observe, label and classify the gamut of sexual experience. New institutions like asylums and prisons, which housed large populations of patients and inmates, furnished physicians with subjects whom they could study. Towards the end of the century, psychiatrists also began to see patients in their own private clinics. "In courts, prisons, hospitals, clinics and private practice, doctors were [now] confronted with the spectacle of criminals and patients exhibiting perverse desires and suffering sexual fixations," writes Stephen Garton. "This was the seedbed for sexology."

During the 1880s and 1890s, a small yet active group of doctors and social reformers began to publish their research. Krafft-Ebing was one of the first to synthesise medical knowledge of sexual perversion. His pioneering *Psychopathia Sexualis* was a compendium of hundreds of what he called "strange cases": men and women who could be aroused only by the touch of silk, the sight of slaughtered animals, or the sensation of being whipped. Some sought sexual satisfaction with children and animals, while others fixated on feet or nostrils. A man with a fetish for hair harassed women on the street by "imprinting" kisses on their heads. (American newspapers reported that several cities were much troubled by such "hair-despoilers".)

Krafft-Ebing defined "perversions" as non-procreative forms of sexuality. Echoing Charles Darwin, who had pointed out a few decades before that humans are animals who are motivated by many of the same instincts of survival, Krafft-Ebing asserted that the purpose of the sexual instinct was "the perpetuation of the species". This was a modern take on an old idea – that the only sexual acts which were "natural" were those that could potentially result in pregnancy – and virtually all sexologists agreed with Krafft-Ebing. Accordingly, any form of sexual behaviour conducted for any reason other than reproduction was deemed abnormal.

He identified four main perversions, coining terms for the first three: sadism, masochism, fetishism and contrary sexual feeling. (The last term was not synonymous with the modern term "homosexual". Krafft-Ebing and most of his colleagues believed that men who experienced contrary sexual feeling, often referred to as "inverts", were attracted to men because they were feminine in character. In today's terms, inverts would be both homosexual and transgender.) By the end of the century, several other taxonomies had been developed but Krafft-Ebing's "eventually set the tone, not only in medical circles but also in everyday life," writes Oosterhuis.

In addition to defining, labelling and classifying sexual deviance, sexologists also attempted to explain it. At first they hypothesised that anatomical defects were to blame. Some thought that enlarged clitorises resulted in lesbianism while Ambroise Tardieu, a prominent French doctor, believed that the shape of the penis and anus determined whether the homosexual played the active or passive role (if the former, he was supposed to have a very thin penis shaped like a dog's; if the latter, a funnel-shaped anus). When the theory that defects of the reproductive organs caused sexual disorders failed to hold up to scrutiny, psychiatrists looked for anomalies in the nervous system and brain. Arguing that the sexual instinct is a function of the cerebral cortex, Krafft-Ebing advanced the idea that the perversion of this instinct was due to lesions on the cortex.

Other doctors believed that it was possible for deviance to be acquired, through wilful perversity or exposure to a disease-ridden social environment like the modern metropolis. Psychiatrists in thrall to the influential, late-19th-century theory of degeneration believed that once such a perversion was picked up, it could be inherited by future generations. This theory posited that one's environment and behaviour could affect one's reproductive cells, so that characteristics acquired in one's lifetime could be transmitted to future generations. According to this view, in the words of one American physician, "Men and women who seek, from mere satiety, variations of the normal method of sexual gratification, stamp their nervous systems with a malign influence which in the next generation may present itself as a true sexual perversion." Any individual whose sexual instincts were "tainted" by hereditary degeneration could be led astray.

In the 1880s, some French and German specialists began to shift their emphasis from biological, physiological and hereditary explanations of deviance to psychological ones. Tardieu was wrong, they said: perversions could not be detected in a specific tissue or organ. Nor could they be acquired, as defenders of degeneration had it. They argued that perversions were involuntary symptoms of psychological disorders. Once understood as "choices" made by the sinful or immoral, perversions were now increasingly perceived as illnesses of the mind over which the sick had no control.

For centuries, sexually transgressive behaviour had been understood as a temporary deviation from the norm. Now sexologists conceived of sexual deviance as a pathological state of being. This theory of perversion inspired psychiatrists to shift their focus from the sexual act itself to the type of individual who carried it out. Accordingly, sexologists created an entirely new nomenclature for the species of deviants they discovered, from the "fetishist" to the "transvestite". This broke with past methods of conceptualising sexuality, notes McLaren:

> Since classical times pretty much the whole range of sexual *practices* had been categorised, but in the late 19th century certain sorts of *persons* – the homosexual, the masochist, the sadist – were discovered or, one might say, invented.

As the discourse of perversion produced by sexology became increasingly influential in the early 20th century, patients began to see in themselves the sexual types sexologists had invented to describe them. After all, "being seen to be a kind of person, or to do a certain kind of act, may affect someone," notes Ian Hacking. Some patients began to call themselves "homosexuals", a word which had been invented in 1869 by a German-Hungarian defender of same-sex love, Karl Maria Kertbeny, and which would eventually be popularised by Krafft-Ebing. Those who saw themselves as homosexual did not necessarily think of themselves as perverted or ill.

In patients' self-conscious assertion of their sexual identities we can detect the emergence of the modern concept of "sexuality". As understandings of perversions evolved over the course of the 19th century, the definition of sexuality shifted. In the first half of the 1800s, the term was primarily used to indicate whether an individual belonged to the male or female sex, and doctors looked to abnormalities in the anatomy to explain sexual deviance. As sexologists shifted their focus from anatomy to psychology, sexuality increasingly became a matter of impulses, tastes and psychic qualities. "Not only the body, but also the personality began to be understood as being completely saturated with sex and sexuality," writes Oosterhuis. Psychiatrists increasingly believed that sexuality determined one's personality. In Krafft-Ebing's *Text-book of Insanity*, published nearly 20 years after *Psychopathia*, he writes, "These anomalies are very important elementary disturbances, since upon the nature of sexual sensibility the mental individuality in greater part depends." Historian Arnold Davidson puts it more succinctly: "To know a person's sexuality is to know that person."

***

In the early 20th century, the idea that normal people should pursue sexual satisfaction began to grip the public imagination. "Sexual love is undoubtedly one of the chief things in life," Sigmund Freud wrote in 1908. Before, a lacklustre sex life might have been shrugged off as another one of life's many minor misfortunes. But in the age of factories, offices and the division of labour, a time when work had become more routine and less fulfilling, members of the middle class made up for their dreary professional lives by adopting the idea that their authentic selves could thrive only in the private sphere. A successful sex and family life was now essential for well-being; many commentators declared that everyone had to experience sensual bliss. "Apart from a few queer fanatics," continued Freud, "all the world knows this and conducts its life accordingly; science alone is too delicate to admit it."

Today, Freud is most famous for founding psychoanalysis, which became the most influential clinical theory and method for the treatment of neuroses of the 20th century. But when he was developing his ideas in fin de siècle Vienna, he was best known as a sexologist. While Krafft-Ebing and others were studying the sexual manias of disturbed criminals and luna-

Left: So committed was Marie Bonaparte to Freud's definition of healthy female sexuality that she had an operation to move her clitoris to the entrance of her vagina, making it possible, she claimed, to have vaginal orgasms

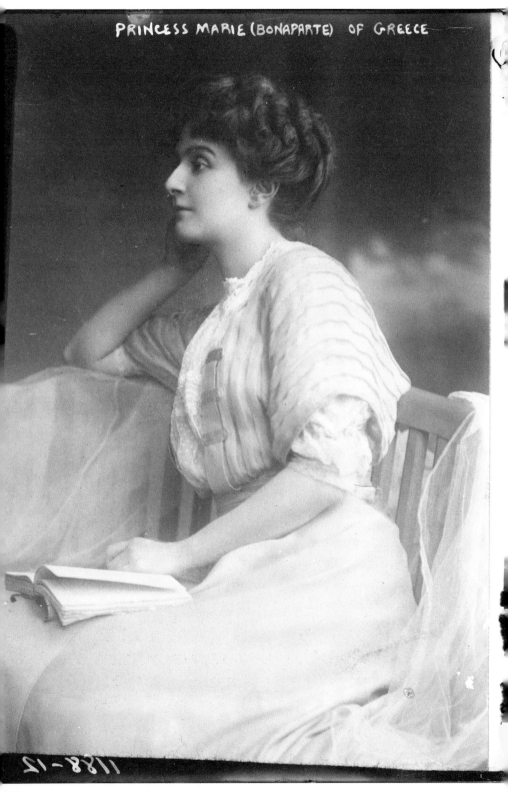

PRINCESS MARIE (BONAPARTE) OF GREECE

1188-12

tics, Freud began to take on respectable neurotics as patients. There was growing demand for his services. As sexual problems came to be seen as serious, open-minded members of the middle class began to direct their concerns not to churchmen or family members but to qualified medical experts who were fluent in the language of science. By treating regular people in addition to perverts, Freud expanded the scope of sexology, making "normal" sexuality the subject of scientific enquiry. This was his "most lasting contribution", in the opinion of McLaren. But rather than underscore the line drawn by sexologists dividing normal from abnormal sexualities, his ideas would blur it.

Freud believed that sexuality was the fundamental cause of neurosis. According to his theory of the mind, the ego ensures – a bit like an engineer – that primitive, unconscious "drives" are, like streams of water, channelled down the correct course. But if the engineer dams or represses the "most unruly of all the instincts" – the sexual instinct – it could burst into the wrong places, causing neuroses.

Freud's definition of the sexual instinct was very different from the sexologists'. As we have seen, they believed that it was a biological urge to procreate. To Freud, the physical throb of lust was accompanied by a complicated stew of emotions in which sensuality mixed with anger, affection and attachment. These emotions did not develop during puberty, as the sexologists had it, but in childhood. When infants sucked their thumbs or explored their genitals, they were expressing what Freud called a "polymorphous perversity". The very idea of infantile sexuality was shocking. As Victorians had fewer and fewer children, it became possible for parents to invest more time and emotion in their relationships with their offspring. Increasingly, middle-class commentators characterised childhood as an age of innocence that ought to be protected. "[Children] were to stay firmly in Eden, with their hands off the apples and deaf to the serpents", as J.H. Plumb put it. Freud scandalised the respectable by arguing that humans first tasted the forbidden fruit in infancy.

Freud would deeply unsettle polite society and his colleagues once again with his claim that children did not necessarily mature into heterosexuals. Sexologists thought it obvious that humans naturally sought to have intercourse with members of the opposite sex. Freud invoked examples from history to prove them wrong: if homosexuality was "unnatural", why was it a veritable institution in ancient Greece? In his analysis he introduced two terms, "sexual object" and "sexual aim": the object referred to the individual to whom one's sexual attentions were directed, the aim referred to how those attentions were expressed (ie, coitus, anal sex, etc). Previous theorists had not distinguished between aim and object. They assumed that the sexual instinct naturally expressed itself through the insertion of the penis into the vagina during intercourse. In what would be his most important insight, Freud declared that object and aim were not fused together. Because the instinct to have sex was not welded to any particular object, "all humans are capable of making a homosexual object choice". This idea seemed to erase altogether the line dividing normal sexuality from abnormal.

The idea that homosexuality was naturally latent in everyone was radical. Teetering on the precipice of revolution, Freud then scurried back from the edge. Homosexuality was natural but he did not, all the same, think it desirable or normal. Healthy humans were heterosexual, he declared.

The trouble was, they weren't inevitably so. The journey towards heterosexuality began in childhood. The emotions of infantile polymorphous perversity had to attach to a love object – normally the mother. In boys, heterosexuality was the result of overcoming the Oedipal complex. It wasn't so simple for girls. Freud characterised the clitoris as the female penis and attributed a "wholly masculine character" to little girls who masturbated. When the "pursuit of pleasure comes under the sway of the reproductive function", girls had to transfer their sexual focus from their clitoris to their vagina. Women who masturbated were therefore "masculine" and suffering from "penis envy". (It was common knowledge among 19th-century doctors that the vagina had few nerve endings. Freud claimed to have discovered the "vaginal orgasm" but in fact he invented it. No matter: the idea that women who did not experience vaginal orgasm were "frigid" soon became widely accepted.)

Forever at risk of toppling over into perversion, heterosexuality was clearly far more fragile than the first sexologists thought. But Freud believed he could cure perversion with psychoanalysis, a form of talking therapy in which the patient confesses his sexual secrets to the trained analyst. Freud's ideas would become highly influential in the first half of the 20th century, particularly in the US. He was by no means universally popular, however. The muddled idea that the grotesque speculations of academics like Freud threatened to corrupt "healthy" sexuality soon became commonplace. Such fears would later be exploited by the authoritarian leaders of the inter-war period.

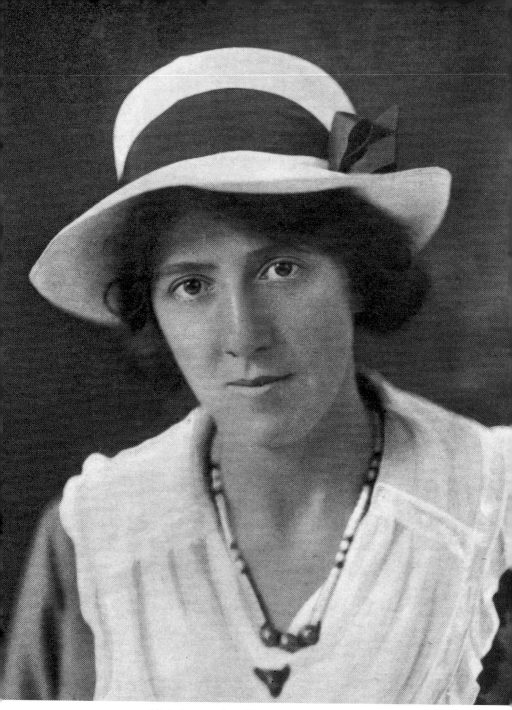

Marie Stopes, author of the sensational sex manual,
Married Love, *published in 1918*

CHAPTER SEVEN

SEXPERTS: BETWEEN THE WARS

In 1916 Marie Stopes, a British scientist, sent the manuscript of her book, *Married Love*, to a prominent radical named Edward Carpenter. He was impressed. The book, he told her, would "terrify Mrs Grundy". The poor woman was already in a bit of a state. The First World War seemed to be attacking everything she stood for. As men departed for the front, women responded to the ensuing labour shortages by abandoning their "rightful place" in the home to work as plumbers, bus conductors, factory hands, civil servants, nurses and doctors. Fears that women would cast off their propriety, just as they had slipped out of their Edwardian skirts to enter the workforce, seemed to be confirmed by sensational reports that women were jumping into bed with young men on their way to the front. Many observed that women were behaving more like men, while the soldiers who returned from the war, shell-shocked and wounded, seemed dangerously emasculated.

It would, however, take more than a war to finish off Mrs Grundy. Fears that the war had encouraged widespread promiscuity were overblown; sexual mores remained recognisably Victorian. The war did foster a climate in which government officials and experts could discuss sexuality more openly than ever before, in the context of improving the health and racial purity of the population, but for most, the subject of sex remained taboo – so much so that the sixth edition of TH Huxley's *Human Physiology* (1915) did not include any reference to the human reproductive system. Ignorance of the facts of life remained widespread, particularly among women. One English nurse recollected that "at 26 years of age [in 1914], I was as ignorant as it was possible to be...Even when I started my midwifery training I never thought fathers had anything to do with it."

Marie Stopes was no better informed. The child of a suffragist who, like many of the first feminists, advocated sexual purity, Stopes was, she said, entirely ignorant of sexual matters when she got married in 1911. But when after five years of marriage she discovered what sexual intercourse actually involved and realised that, thanks to her husband's impotence, she was still a virgin, Stopes went to the British Museum in London. There, in the restricted-access section, she read almost every scholarly work and medical account of sexual theory and practice. A paleobotanist by training, Stopes had already published many academic papers. To spare other women her "years of heartache and blind questioning in the dark", she decided to write a book for young husbands and "all those who are betrothed in love" about "the supreme human art": sex. One month after some British women were given the right to vote in February 1918, *Married Love* was published. A book that made Victorian husbands gasp, according to Stopes, it would help to usher in a new sexual era.

The primary argument of *Married Love* was that women, far from being passionless, felt the burn of desire as intensely as men, and that wives had as much right to sexual satisfaction as their husbands. The trouble was that sexual ignorance was endemic. Many brides, almost entirely in the dark about what married life entailed, greeted with "horror" the first night of marriage, particularly if their eager grooms were boorish, selfish or uneducated about sex. Radically for her time, Stopes believed that this was a problem. The stability of society relied on the stability of marriage and the stability of marriage, she argued, relied on the sexual fulfilment of both husband *and* wife. So she endeavoured to teach husbands how to arouse their wives' dormant passions. While marriage manuals published before 1918 avoided mentioning intercourse directly, *Married Love* explicitly described the act of coitus as well as male and female physiology and anatomy. It drove home the point that it was a man's duty to behave like a lover and pleasure his wife so that they climaxed together.

To achieve marital bliss, men were going to have to make some sacrifices. Stopes argued that the husband must relinquish his ancient conjugal right, which permitted a man to have sex with his wife on demand. Too often, he exercised this right at the expense of his wife's pleasure, Stopes wrote, so he was to restrain himself until her desire was at its peak. That might happen just once or twice a month. Stopes believed that desire moved through men and women at different rhythms: "man's desire naturally wells up every day or every few days, and woman's only every fortnight or every month". If her desire was reaching its zenith, he was to "woo" her. But if his courtship failed, he was to deny himself until she also desired sexual intercourse. That could mean waiting a couple of weeks. On no account was he to turn elsewhere – to a prostitute or mistress – for sexual relief while he waited, for the bond between husband and wife was sacred.

Stopes's challenge to husbands was radical – it assumed that men could control behaviour that had been assumed to be instinctual – though not a new one. The first generation of feminists in Britain and America had condemned the male conjugal right. Accepting society's belief that women were passionless, they argued that men should learn to control their animal urges rather than debase women with their brutish advances. This implied, according to Stopes, "that sex-life is a low, physical and degrading necessity which a pure woman is above enjoying". It did not have to be that way, she argued. Equipped with the right know-how, a couple could transform sex into a "glorious unfolding", one that a woman of virtue could delight in, and should, for regular sexual intercourse was essential to women's physical health, Stopes claimed. She did not want men to embrace chastity, as the feminists urged; she wanted them to sexually satisfy their wives.

Married Love was a sensation, eventually selling more than a million copies. Stopes, who would go on to become a celebrated women's rights campaigner and eugenicist, received thousands of letters from readers, thanking her for enlightening them. "It is books like yours", one wrote, "that are needed to clear away the old evil conspiracy of secrecy which has ruined so many women's lives." Stopes was by no means the first to break Mrs Grundy's vow of silence. In the late 19th century, sexologists investigated sexual perversions, eugenicists advocated the public management of reproduction and, a few decades later, reformers began to campaign for the liberalisation of sex-crime laws. But ordinary people still did not talk about sex. Plenty of them did, however, read *Married Love*, along with much of the new literature on marital sexuality it inspired. *Ideal Marriage*, a sex manual written by Theodoor van de Velde, a Dutch physician, in 1926, was the most popular book of the inter-war period and would be translated into every European language.

The genre's success stemmed from its positive, romantic portrayal of intercourse. The prevailing view held it to be a vile expression of an animal instinct, but van de Velde, for instance, celebrated it as a loving "communion" in which a couple's "souls meet and touch as do their bodies". And though their insistence that women had a right to sexual satisfaction was radical, authors defended family life and conventional gender roles. Stopes was critical of husbands but assumed that men were innately aggressive and women passive, while Van de Velde took it as a given that brides would be virgins and new husbands sexually experienced.

Readers of *Married Love* were disappointed only by Stopes's omission of any information about reproduction. Like those who followed in her wake, she sought to disassociate the pleasures of sex from childbearing, but many of her female correspondents informed her that they could not give themselves over to the "glorious unfolding" for fear they might conceive. Realising that her dream of female sexual fulfilment would not become a reality until women could limit their fertility, she resolved to campaign for better education and access to contraception.

Stopes was entering a crowded field: Malthus and his disciples, the neo-Malthusians, had long argued for curbing fertility on the economic grounds that the population would outstrip the food supply if it grew unchecked, while sexual radicals extolled contraception as the key to unlocking free love. Aware that birth control's association with radicalism made it seem like a threat to the moral order, Stopes and Margaret Sanger, an American feminist, sought to frame family limitation as not just economically but morally imperative. To that end, they "developed the positive argument that contraception was not only compatible with pleasure but essential if the woman's passions were to be allowed full expression", notes McLaren. With her characteristic energy, Stopes wrote another advice manual, on contraception, just months after *Married Love* was published, and opened

Britain's first birth-control clinic in London in 1921.

***

Most Europeans and Americans, of course, did not read sex manuals. But long-term, structural changes to the family created the conditions necessary for the realisation of Stopes's goal: the eroticisation of the bond between husband and wife. The fertility rate, which began to decline in the 19th century, more than halved between the turn of the century and the Second World War. Small, two-child families became the norm.

As birth control became increasingly socially acceptable, thanks in part to the evangelisation of Stopes and Sanger, it began to be adopted by the middle classes. By the 1920s, contraception was widely used in Germany, where birth control was legal and dispensed via an extensive network of sexual advice clinics. In 1936, American doctors were legally permitted to prescribe contraceptives, and growing numbers of white, middle-class women began to use the diaphragm. Western families were becoming smaller, more mobile and less tied down by clan relationships. The emergence of the nuclear family gave middle-class couples more time to invest in each other. As it became increasingly possible to disentangle sex from reproduction, many gradually embraced the notion that husbands and wives should treat each other like lovers.

It was a novel idea. The Victorians had romanticised sex as a spiritual union whose goal was conception; the ideal wife never felt the itch of desire. But in the early 20th century, some women began to challenge the image of the pure Victorian wife by stepping out of the private sphere and into the public. In the 1910s, single women from the elite who wore daring "flapper" outfits started going to restaurants and cabarets without the supervision of chaperones. They weren't the first to have a visible presence outside of the home – 19th-century suffragists, social purists and philanthropists had produced a less-exclusively domestic image of women – but they did flout Victorian gender norms in a highly public manner.

Some commentators worried that the New Woman, as she was called, posed a threat to marriage. As she became increasingly economically independent – many women were getting jobs as secretaries, teachers and shop girls – and mingled with men in the new dance halls and picture palaces, she seemed to be losing interest in marriage. Experts sought to make matrimony more appealing to the fun-loving New Woman by redefining it as a relationship whose primary purpose was sexual pleasure and companionship rather than children or duty. "Sex, once seen as potentially threatening to family life, was now presented as its glue," writes McLaren. Manuals like *Ideal Marriage* told men to arouse their partners through clitoral stimulation; van de Velde even advocated the "genital kiss" (oral sex). The figure of the passionless Victorian wife was gradually making way for the modern sensual partner.

With greater access to birth control, more knowledge about sex, and a new cultural ideal that prized mutual sexual satisfaction in marriage, did couples have better sex? Surveys indicate that there was some improvement. Less than 40 percent of German women born between 1895 and 1907 had ever had an orgasm, according to one study, while 78 percent of those born between 1907 and 1916 had. A majority of American women born in the late 19th century never reached orgasm during intercourse while a majority of women born in the 1920s almost always achieved it. The latter also experimented with a greater variety of sexual acts, oral sex among them. Alfred Kinsey, an American scientist who conducted the survey, attributed this shift in female responsiveness to more forthright attitudes and greater premarital experience among young women. Young middle-class couples, it seemed, had made great strides towards the ideal of companionate marriage.

The picture was very different for working-class women. It remained difficult for them to access reliable methods of birth control or information about sex. Living in crowded rooms with no privacy, young couples couldn't very well indulge in the leisurely foreplay recommended by manual authors. For most people, sexual pleasure was ultimately less important than the social status and economic security conferred by marriage. "Whatever the problems they encountered in marriage," writes Jeffrey Weeks, "it meant public acceptance, a division of labour that ensured women's economic and social survival, and legitimate children. For most people sexual pleasure was secondary to that."

***

Suspicions of lesbians grew after the war. This was new. The Victorian ideology of separate spheres had encouraged affection between women.

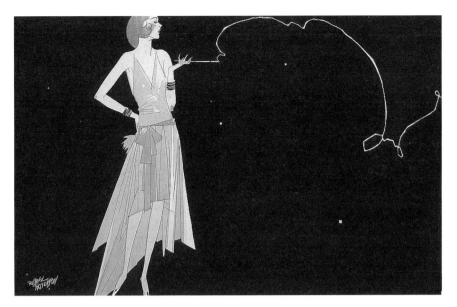

*"Where there's smoke there's fire": An illustration of a fashionably dressed
flapper drawn by Russell Patterson in the 1920s*

Behaviour that we today might consider an expression of lesbian desire –
young women embracing, kissing and sharing beds – was condoned, even
recommended. Victorian doctors regarded emotional relationships between
young women as a passing phase that would prepare them for their sex lives
with men. Though some women never grew out of this phase, experts did
not think that what female lovers did together could be considered sexual.
The prevailing view of female sexuality held that it was activated by the
maternal instinct or the stimulation of the male. Many were perplexed by
the idea that it could exist independently of the urge to mate and reproduce,
if they encountered this idea at all. Lesbianism figured so little in the public
imagination that an effort to have it criminalised in Britain in 1921 failed
because almost nobody knew what it was, according to Lord Desart, who
challenged the bill in Parliament:

You are going to tell the whole world that there is such an offence,
to bring it to the notice of women who have never heard of it, never
thought of it, never dreamt of it. I think that is a very great mis-
chief.

Of course, sexologists were familiar with lesbians (Havelock Ellis's wife was one) but they were focused on what they regarded as the most serious sexual problems: perversions associated with the failure of male arousal.

As Western culture began to eroticise marriage in the inter-war period, however, same-sex infatuations started to be treated with misgiving. Reformers who championed companionate marriages looked down their noses at female intimacy. Such "women can only play with each other", Stopes sneered; they could never have "real", i.e. heterosexual, relationships. While most sexologists believed by the early 20th century that homosexuality could not be prevented in men because it was inborn, there was confusion about the nature of lesbianism. American doctors linked it both to the anatomical abnormality of a large clitoris and to acquired habits, like masturbation and masculine hobbies. Stopes believed that while a few women were innately lesbian, most "drifted into it lazily or out of curiosity". The fear that women could be seduced into lesbianism seeped into popular culture. Novels featured spinster lesbians leading innocent young girls astray. In *La Garçonne*, a best-selling French novel published in 1922, the predatory Lady Springfield inveigles the innocent young heroine to a lesbian orgy in a brothel.

It was in this climate of growing suspicion that Radclyffe Hall, an English novelist, gained notoriety in the 1920s, first for her dapper masculine appearance (she sported short hair, smoking jackets and a monocle), then for her novel, *The Well of Loneliness*. Published in 1928, it made a splash by defending lesbianism. The heroine, Stephen, is confused by the direction of her desire until she discovers a battered old book by Krafft-Ebing in her father's locked bookcase. "God's cruel," she exclaims after reading it. "He let us get flawed in the making." Echoing Krafft-Ebing, who thought that lesbianism was innate and expressed through masculine physical features, Hall gave Stephen narrow hips and broad shoulders – flesh-and-blood expressions of a lesbian nature the wretched Stephen abhors but cannot deny. This characterisation of lesbianism as inborn undercut the idea that women like Stephen could be "fixed" or should be punished.

Hall's failure to criticise lesbianism led to the prosecution of the book, which was eventually banned in England after 1929. Yet the publicity surrounding the trial advertised lesbianism, just as Wilde's trial had drawn attention to homosexuality. The women invoked by Lord Desart in 1921 – the "women who have never heard of it, never thought of it, never

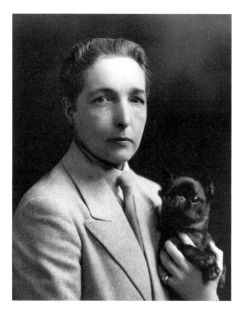

Radclyffe Hall, author of
The Well of Loneliness *(1928)*

dreamt of it" – now certainly had heard of it, thought of it and maybe even dreamt of it. Over 5,000 women wrote to Hall. Many recognised themselves in Stephen and were now able to put their inchoate feelings into words.

Female readers who corresponded with Hall often wanted to know where they might meet other women like them. At the time, lesbian communities were nascent. Before the 20th century, most women did not have independent financial means, severely restricting their behaviour, but as women began to find employment in factories and the service industry, they gained a measure of independence. Accordingly, lesbian subcultures began to emerge in New York, in Greenwich Village, and Paris, in the aristocratic and artistic circles of Colette, Renée Vivien, Natalie Clifford Barney and Gertrude Stein. The culture was most developed in Berlin, the capital city of inter-war lesbianism. As Anna Clark notes, "the modern Berlin lesbian – perhaps a doctor, a shop girl, a typist – could entertain friends or live with a lover in her chic apartment, leaf through several lesbian magazines, and saunter out to a different lesbian club each night" (one was called the Café Dorian Grey). At lesbian bars women could add

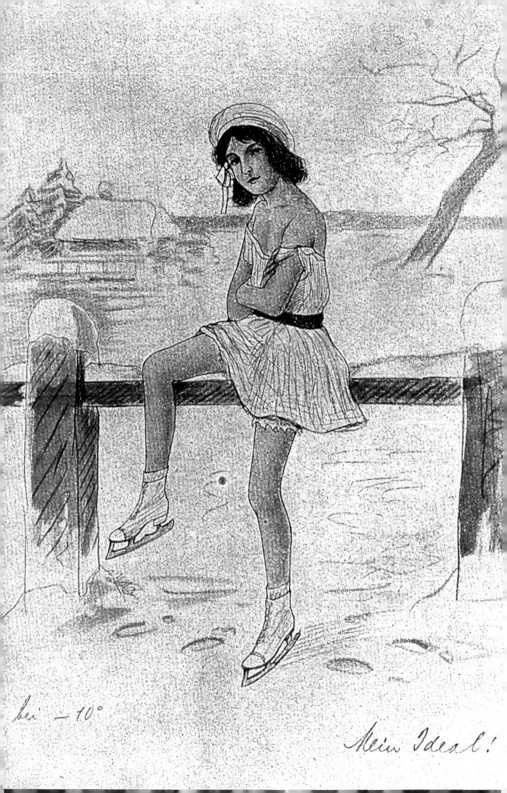

bei −10°

Mein Ideal!

their two cents to the debates about the nature of lesbian identity held by magazines like *The Friend* or *Garçonne*. Some agreed with the sexologists' claim that lesbians were masculine inverts, a view which was common among the British public, which associated lesbianism with a masculine appearance after the *The Well of Loneliness* trial. But others critiqued this idea. They pointed out that in addition to the masculine "bubi" or butch figure there was the feminine "gamine" and repudiated the notion that the latter were only superficially lesbian.

***

Traditional Germans were appalled and frightened by what they saw as the decadence of the Weimar Republic, with its cabarets, gay and lesbian clubs and birth-control clinics. As the Great Depression sowed economic misery in the early 1930s, with 40 percent unemployment and long queues for bread, Adolf Hitler gained popular support on the right by exploiting widespread political and economic concerns and by promising to purge Germany of sexual decadence. This policy was central to his doctrine of the master race. Hitler believed that the Germanic people – whom he called "Aryans" and vaunted for their virility – were superior to all others, and that their racial purity must remain inviolate. He identified and condemned certain types of people who threatened to contaminate the Aryan race (Jews, Roma, the disabled) or frustrate its growth (homosexuals, because they had non-reproductive sex, and women who wanted small families).

When the Nazis came to power in January 1933, Hitler began to deliver on his promise. The Nazis shuttered gay bars and birth-control clinics, revoked the medical-necessity clause for abortion and suppressed the sex-reform movement, trashing sexologist Magnus Hirschfeld's Institute for Sexual Research and burning his collection of over 10,000 books. In July 1933, Hitler went a step further: he legalised the forced sterilisation of the deaf, blind, mentally ill and anyone else doctors deemed "unworthy of life".

With the benefit of hindsight it is evident that in passing such a measure Nazi Germany was embarking on a journey that would end with the extermination of millions of non-Aryans in concentration camps. But in 1933, few envisioned such horrors. Many in the West actually considered sterilisation a compassionate, sensible method for ensuring undesirables

Left: Among the types of sexual pathology catalogued by sexologist Magnus Hirschfeld was a fetish for the cold, illustrated here (1921)

did not reproduce.

That they did was thanks to an English scientist named Francis Galton. In the late 19th century, most Darwinians thought that natural selection would lead inevitably to the improvement of the human race. But Galton couldn't help noticing that the lower classes – people of "poor breeding" – were reproducing in greater numbers than the middle-class, whose members were increasingly using contraception. Galton inferred that the struggle for survival was being won by the unfit, but he believed that their victory could be thwarted by "eugenics", the science of improving a population by managing breeding. He and his followers hoped that states would adopt a carrot-and-stick approach, by on the one hand providing child allowances, for instance, to encourage the reproduction of those deemed "healthy", and on the other, restraining the reproduction of the "unhealthy" by institutionalising or sterilising them.

By the early 20th century, eugenics had found a wide range of prominent European and American supporters, from feminists (Margaret Sanger), doctors (Auguste Forel) and sexologists (Havelock Ellis, Marie Stopes) to politicians on both the left and right. Eugenicists seeking to translate their ideas into government policy found greatest success in the United States. By stoking fears of "race suicide" (ie, that the number of blacks and immigrants would exceed the number of WASPs), the eugenics lobby would create the most vigorous sterilisation programme of the early 20th century. In 1907, Indiana passed the world's first law sanctioning surgeries for the "feeble-minded". By the late 1930s, California – the most ardently eugenic of the 50 states – had operated on over 20,000 patients.

Eugenicists did not meet with approval everywhere. The Vatican prohibited any form of birth control so Catholic Europe refused to legalise sterilisation. Though many in Britain did not want the country to be "swamped with imbeciles", ultimately the government thought surgery too harsh a measure. Most of the other nations of Protestant Europe, however, had no such qualms and joined the United States in establishing sterilisation programmes. Sixty-thousand Swedish citizens would be operated on between 1935 and 1976.

By the time the Nazis unfurled their swastika flags from the Reichstag, sterilisation had been discussed in Germany for years. Once the Nazis were in power, they mandated the sterilisation of the mentally and physically impaired, modelling their programme on America's. They didn't stop there. In 1935, Hitler passed a succession of laws that tightened his grip

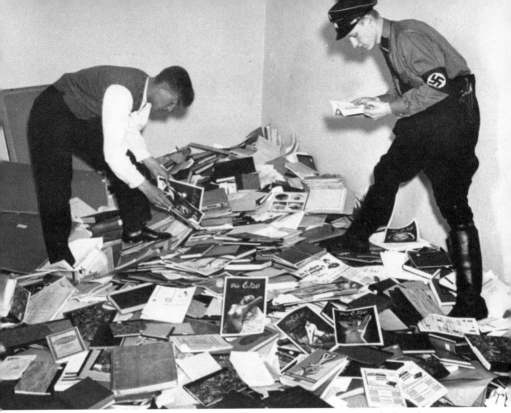

May, 1933. Nazi Stormtroopers ransack Magnus Hirschfeld's Institute for Sexual Research in Berlin. These books were carted off to be burnt

on Germans' bodies. He forbade Jews and Aryans from having sex or marrying each other and criminalised not just "unnatural" intercourse but all sexual contact between men. He also re-legalised abortion in certain cases so that the Nazis could force the termination of pregnancies among prostitutes, the promiscuous, the mentally disabled, Jews, German women carrying the children of Jewish men, and foreign slaver workers. As McLaren points out, there were politicians in every Western state who were concerned about the mixing of races but "the Nazis went furthest in their remedies", eventually sterilising 400,000 Germans, forcing 100,000 women to get abortions, and sending between 5,000 and 15,000 men convicted of homosexuality to concentration camps. The Nazis sought total control over sex and reproduction and, in many cases, secured it. Sterilisations led on to euthanasia and euthanasia culminated in Hitler's final solution: genocide.

CHAPTER EIGHT

SEXUAL REVOLUTION

During the Second World War, drawings and photographs of pin-up girls like Betty Grable kept lonely American GIs company in their barracks. When the war ended and soldiers went home, it would not be long before they discovered a new genre of magazine that would cater to their hankering for pneumatic blondes. The first issue of *Playboy* went on sale in December 1953. Marilyn Monroe was on the cover and in the centrefold, this time nude. "We aren't a 'family magazine'," winked the introductory note.

Playboy wasn't the first men's mag to titillate its readers with bosomy babes but its brazenness, according to one reviewer, "makes old issues of *Esquire*, in its most uninhibited days, look like trade bulletins from the Woman's Christian Temperance Union". Accompanying the nude photographs was a philosophy of life, the greatest exponent of which was the magazine's founder, Hugh Hefner. The naked women in *Playboy* weren't mere pin-ups, he said, they were "a triumph of sexuality, an end of Puritanism". Hefner wanted to remove the obstacles impeding the free expression

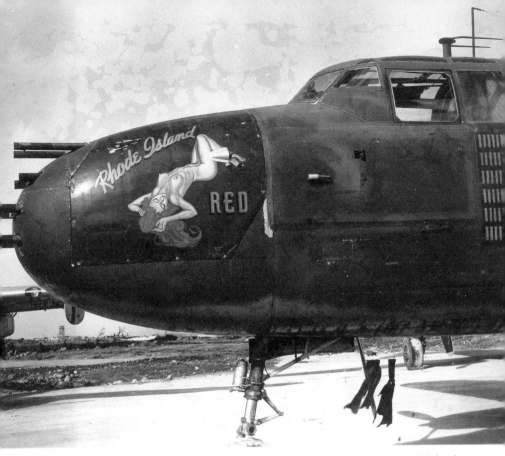

During the Second World War, fighter planes like this B25 bomber were sometimes decorated with female nudes. The US Navy hoped that "nose art" would boost morale

of male sexuality – marriage among them. *Playboy* described husbands as "sorry, regimented" creatures shackled to domineering, spendthrift wives. Bachelors were to forget marriage, "enjoy the pleasures the female has to offer without becoming emotionally involved", and spend their money on luxurious lifestyles – just like Hefner did. With circulation surpassing the million mark by 1960, the magazine made him rich. In 1959, he moved into a 48-room mansion in Chicago. He needed a place big enough to accommodate all thirty of his *Playboy* "bunny" housemates.

Hefner's slick critique of marriage and family came at a time when those institutions had never seemed more robust. After the Depression and the war sent shock waves through daily life, Americans and Europeans responded by energetically shoring up the family as the foundation for social stability. In the age of the baby boom, English and American women married earlier, had their children sooner, and had more of them. Television shows like *The Adventures of Ozzie and Harriet*, an American sitcom, provided a model for family life and gender relations that seemed to guarantee domestic harmony. Ozzie was a successful, white-collar worker, Harriet was a homemaker, and with their sons they lived in a sub-urban house equipped with kitchen appliances, a washing machine and, of course, a television. As the affluent American middle class joined Ozzie and Harriet in the suburbs, they brought with them their parents' sexual mores. A good sex life was essential to one's happiness and the health of a marriage not because it led to children per se but because it was mutually pleasurable. It went without saying that sex was only permissible between a man and a woman who were husband and wife – though affianced lovers who went all the way were tolerated.

Anyone who switched on the evening news, however, would have scoffed at the suggestion that this was the "golden age of the family". As America plunged into the Cold War, fears about the ability of the country and the family to stand firm against its enemies proliferated. Just as Senator Joseph McCarthy declared that Communists were infiltrating the government, his Republican colleagues raised the spectre of homosexuals infiltrating families and seducing impressionable youths into deviance. But even as local police forces responded to the "homosexual menace" by making sweeping arrests in gay neighbourhoods, middle-class families increasingly seemed to be battling agents of subversion on the home front. Teenagers flouted rules of sexual decorum by channelling the smouldering sensuality of idols like Elvis Presley. Women who were discontented with their roles as wives and mothers sought help from psychoanalysts, who tried to coax them back to femininity. Men who complained that their wives were too independent increasingly sought refuge from their families in the warm embrace of *Playboy* centrefolds.

Many American churches, citizen groups and politicians could not stand the fact that magazines like *Playboy*, which undermined the family, were openly sold on newsstands. From the mid-1930s to the 1950s, they sought to reinvigorate 19th-century laws which prohibited the public display of sexuality, laws which had been progressively weakened since the First World War. Focused as they were on scrubbing the filth out of popular culture, these moralists were blindsided when, in 1948, a respectable scien-

PLAYBOY

ENTERTAINMENT FOR **MEN**

50c

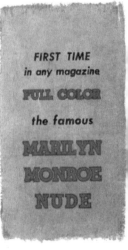

FIRST TIME
in any magazine

FULL COLOR

the famous

**MARILYN
MONROE
NUDE**

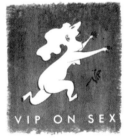

VIP ON SEX

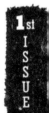

1st
I
S
S
U
E

tist named Alfred Kinsey published *Sexual Behaviour in the Human Male*. This study, and its companion report on "the human female" published five years later, would make sex a topic of public conversation in a way that no previous book or event in the US ever had.

It did not at first glance look like a book that would electrify the nation. Soberly written, the report, which collected data on the sexual behaviour of thousands of ordinary, white American men, was more than 800 pages long and chock-full of charts. But Kinsey's findings were extraordinary. Rejecting the moralising approach of previous sexologists, who categorised sexual behaviour as either normal or abnormal, he simply asked his subjects how they achieved sexual release. Among his male subjects, he discovered that masturbation was ubiquitous, that almost 90 percent had had pre-marital intercourse and that over a third had had at least one homosexual experience. His data on women were similarly revelatory: they indicated that just half were virgins when they married, and that 28 percent had had sexual contact with another female. What the sexologists condemned as "abnormal" behaviour, Kinsey wryly noted, wasn't abnormal at all.

The public reception of the Kinsey reports would help to sweep away the remnants of America's 19th-century obscenity laws. Because Kinsey was a man of science it was safe for the press to cover his work – which it did, extensively. He appeared on the cover of *Time* magazine while his first book spent half a year on the *New York Times* bestseller list. Newspaper editors learned that most readers weren't appalled to see articles about sex in their morning paper. If anything, opinion polls revealed the public wanted to learn more about sex.

This response to Kinsey's studies shaped the climate in which the Supreme Court reviewed Victorian obscenity laws. During the Fifties, moralists' vigorous complaints had spurred local police forces to crack down on pornography. But these purity crusaders – unlike their 19th-century counterparts – did not share the views of the mainstream. The suppression of porn resulted in so much litigation that, by the late 1950s, obscenity cases were flooding the Supreme Court. From 1957-1967, the court gradually narrowed the definition of obscenity until it had effec-tively ruled that sex was appropriate for public consumption. The effect was immediate and profound. Ever-more explicit pornographic magazines, books and films mushroomed while the producers of mainstream media – from Hollywood and television studios to publishing houses and the press – immediately sought to capitalise on the new liberal climate. Sex had once been confined to the private sphere; now it was being released into the public sphere. Similar forces were at work in western Europe. In 1961 and 1964, Britain decriminalised sexually explicit material if it could be proven to have artistic or academic merit. Denmark, Sweken and West Germany decriminalised porn in the late Sixties and early Seventies. As John D'Emilio and Estelle B. Freedman write, "The veil of 19th-century reticence was torn away, as sex was put on display".

***

As they flipped through *Playboy* or gazed at scantily clad women newly plastered on hoardings and adverts, men must have wondered where they might encounter their flesh-and-blood counterparts: women they could take home for no-strings-attached sex. In the Fifties and early Sixties, most young American women saw sex as something they would do once they were married or in a committed relationship. Luckily for would-be playboys, Helen Gurley Brown would persuade many women that they didn't have to treat sex so seriously.

A careerist who would go on to make a commercial success of *Cosmopolitan* magazine as its editor, Brown made her name in 1962 with *Sex and the Single Girl*, a book that served as the *Playboy* for the unattached, working woman. Brown wanted to convince her readers that it wasn't "dirty" to have sex before marriage. Girls can say "yes", she wrote, even "nice, single girls". In fact, they should say "yes" frequently: men are "a lot more fun by the dozen". Sure, get married eventually – but not now. Marriage is "insurance for the *worst* years of your life. During your best years you don't need a husband." You just needed a job to earn the money necessary to live the life of a single girl. Her message resonated: *Sex and the Single Girl* was a best-selling book of the early Sixties.

Hefner and Brown put into words what at least some of America's young, single urbanites were thinking. In the early 1960s, these men and women created a new singles culture, throwing weekend parties that were announced in local newspapers. It was not long before savvy businessmen saw the opportunity in this market of prosperous, sexually available people. Bookstores began to stock guidebooks for the unattached while singles bars opened in cities across the country. Men and women eager to

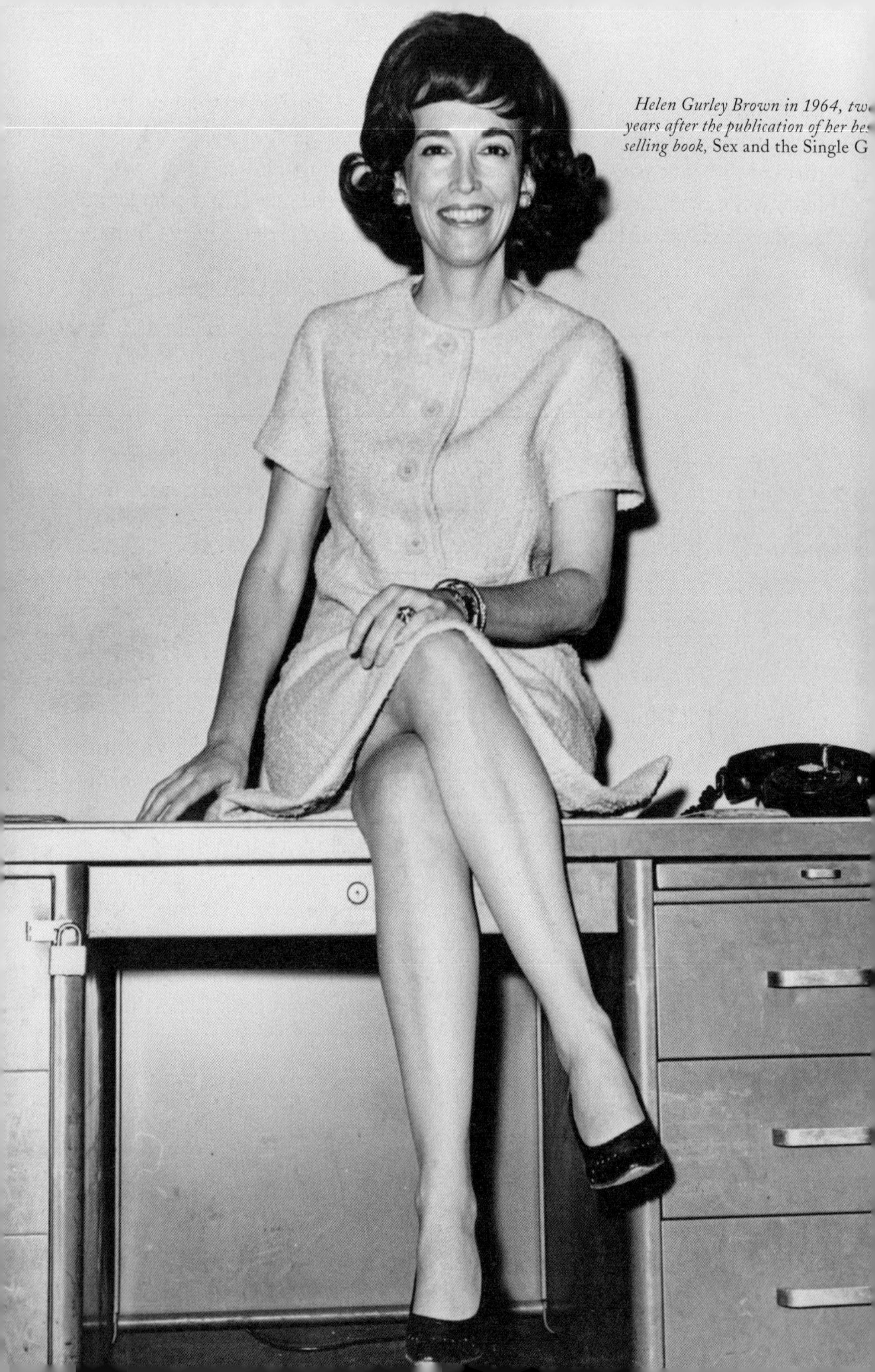

Helen Gurley Brown in 1964, tw
years after the publication of her bes
selling book, Sex and the Single G

meet someone with whom they could have a fling flocked to the new bars. The middle class regarded such singletons not with outrage, as they did turn-of-the-century working-class youths who mingled together in dance halls and movie houses, but with fascination. On the face of it, society still adored Ozzie and Harriet but it envied women like Helen Gurley Brown – and needed her. Built on an ethic of consumption, the post-war economy relied on the single, working woman to spend her disposable income on clothes, cosmetics, home furnishings, party caterers, vacations and cocktails – just as Brown urged.

***

The first major attack on the era's marriage-focused sexual mores was launched in America by entrepreneurs like Hefner and Brown who used sex to sell their products – products which, in their case, encouraged consumers to put off matrimony, perhaps indefinitely, and embrace promiscuity. The second major assault, as D'Emilio and Freedman argue, came from political and cultural radicals who, they said, sought to bring about a "genuine sexual revolution" free of "playboy bromides" uttered by those "false prophets of Eros", Hefner and Brown. White American college students who were inspired by the black civil-rights movement, outraged by the Vietnam war and fearful of the draft, they began to take political action against "the establishment" in the mid-1960s. Coalescing into the New Left, they developed a broad critique of American life, attacking economic inequality, racism, materialism and conventional attitudes to sex. Believing that sexism was a pillar of capitalism, male members of the New Left advocated a free-love morality. "There was a lot of this belief that if you took off your knickers you'd smash the state," recalled one participant.

The cause of free love was taken up with zeal by hippies. Mocking the values of the middle class, "flower children" established communes where they dispensed with the nuclear family along with sexual restraint. A shocked middle America condemned hippie counter-culture. But by the late 1960s, it had caught on among the mainstream. In 1969 hundreds of thousands of youths descended on the town of Woodstock, New York for a weekend of sex, drugs and rock music. As revellers danced naked in fields to the music of Janis Joplin and Jimi Hendrix, it was clear that the counterculture, in concert with consumer culture, had broken with the sexual mores of the past half century. "The old taboos are dead or dying," *Newsweek* observed. "A new, more permissive society is taking shape." Would it devise a new moral code?

***

The year was 1968. Outside a convention hall in Atlantic City, New Jersey, nearly 100 demonstrators gathered, all women. They were picketing the Miss America Pageant. A few months before, mass protests had erupted in New York, Paris, Italy, Poland, West Germany. Now it was the turn of these women. As they tossed bras, girdles, high heels and a copy of *Playboy* into their "freedom trash can", they declared that the only "free" woman is "the woman who is no longer enslaved by ludicrous beauty standards". They belonged, they said, to the Women's Liberation Movement.

The winners of the Miss America pageant embodied some of the traits society most valued in young women: beauty, poise, savoir faire and, as the swimwear competition revealed, a hint of sensuality – qualities of a wife-in-training rather than a bit of skirt. But as Betty Friedan revealed in 1963 with her book, *The Feminine Mystique*, many housewives were deeply discontented. They did not recognise themselves in the idealised figure of the "truly feminine" woman who devoted herself to her family and had no

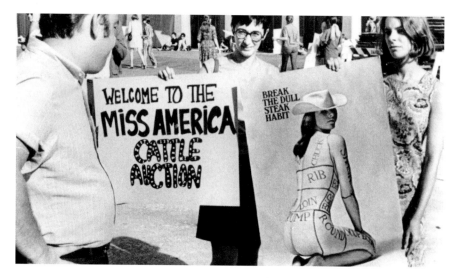

A protest against Miss America in Atlantic City in 1968

desire for higher education or a career. Their dissatisfaction extended into the bedroom. The inter-war ideal of companionate marriage envisioned husband and wife as equals in the bedroom. But men and women often had very different understandings of the meaning of sex: many women associated it with love, men with physical release. And equality in bed meant nothing when one partner was economically dependant on the other.

There were signs in the Sixties that the society which had produced the American housewife was changing. Greater numbers of women were pursuing higher education and they were more likely to see work as an end in itself rather than a stepping stone to marriage. More women joined the work force and in 1964, the Civil Rights Act made it illegal to discriminate against a woman because of her sex. In the mid-Sixties, the Supreme Court removed any prohibitions against the use of contraception, first by married couples, then by the unmarried. The pill, which went on sale in the US in 1960 and in Britain in 1961, changed American and European women's lives. It was inexpensive and easy to use. Women no longer had to rely on men to slip on a condom or practise *coitus interruptus* effectively. The pill put women firmly in control of their fertility and allowed them to sexually experiment. Change was afoot – but it wasn't happening fast enough.

In 1966, Friedan kick-started American second-wave feminism by founding the National Organisation for Women which campaigned to end sexual discrimination. But the movement derived its vitality from a different group of young, radical women who, in 1967, began meeting in groups all around the country for "consciousness-raising" sessions. The idea was to talk about their experiences to help them understand what it meant to be a woman and to develop a feminist perspective on the world. Much of their focus was on sexuality. They discussed the problems of rape, abortion, pornography and sex itself. Denouncing the "myth of the vaginal orgasm", feminists sided with Kinsey and two other American sexologists, William Masters and Virginia Johnson, all of whom had repudiated Freudian theory by identifying the clitoris, rather than the vagina, as the source of the female orgasm. With the rediscovery of the clitoris, separatist feminists began to argue that men were dispensable and that women ought to embrace lesbianism, for political as well as for personal reasons. By the early 1970s the movement had found mouthpieces in *Ms* magazine, edited by Gloria Steinem, and *Spare Rib* in London. Feminists across Western Europe were debating the same matters as their American sisters.

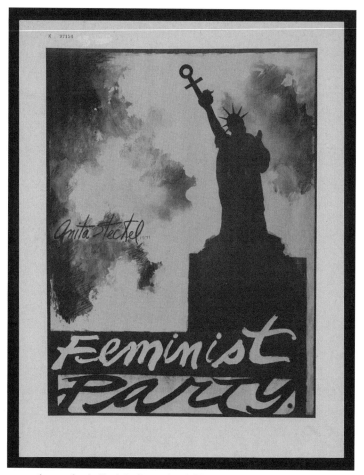

A poster for the Feminist Party, founded in 1971 by one of the instigators of the 1968 Miss America Pageant protest, Florynce Kennedy

It was easy to brand feminists "frigid" and "frustrated", as their opponents did. Most were critical of the way the sexual revolution had transformed sexual freedom for women into "the right that is a duty". But feminists weren't opposed to sex. What they wanted was control over their bodies. At their gatherings, they'd realised that what they'd thought were unique experiences of female helplessness – at the hands of men, doctors, church-men and advertisers – were common to most women. From this realisation sprang the insight that "the personal is political", the theory that their troubling experiences were the consequences of a society that consigned women to an inferior status than men. "In reaching these conclusions, radical women's liberationists laid the foundation for a vastly expanded terrain of politics," write D'Emilio and Freedman. "Marriage, the family and motherhood were reinterpreted as institutions that maintained the oppression of women."

At gatherings like the International Tribunal of Crimes Against Women, held in Brussels, Belgium in 1976, feminists developed critiques of institutions that deprived them of control over their own bodies. Their activism would gradually change minds, customs – even laws. American feminists' most significant achievement was in the realm of reproductive rights. At the time, 19th-century statutes criminalising abortion were still on the books in many states, and hundreds of thousands of women resorted to back-alley abortions. Feminists believed that women would never gain full equality with men until they had absolute control over their fertility. They recast the debate about abortion in terms of women's "rights" over their own bodies. When, in 1973, the Supreme Court heard the case of Roe v Wade, it ruled that it was a women's constitutional right to have an abortion in the first trimester. It was the movement's most dramatic victory.

***

Before the decade was out, one last radical cause would emerge from the "youth rebellion". On a Friday night in June 1969, the Manhattan police raided a gay bar in Greenwich Village. During the Sixties, gay venues were routinely shut down but this time the patrons of the Stonewall Inn refused to leave. A fight broke out and "the scene became explosive", reported the *Village Voice*. "Almost by signal the crowd erupted into cobblestone and bottle heaving." The rioting lasted the whole weekend. Those who later returned found the slogan "Gay Power" graffitied all over the neighbourhood. It was a declaration of intent. Within weeks, gay and lesbian New Yorkers had formed the Gay Liberation Front, an organisation that styled itself on the revolutionary New Left and sought justice for homosexuals.

Thanks to the growth of gay and lesbian subcultures during the 1950s and 1960s, a more relaxed attitude about the public discussion of homosexuality, and anger over police persecution, the GLF's rallying cries of "gay power" were quickly taken up beyond New York and the US. In Britain, which had decriminalised gay sex in 1967, an organisation directly modelled on the GLF launched in 1971. Similar lesbian and gay liberation movements emerged in other Western European nations in the early 1970s. Far from thinking of homosexuality as an abnormality, the GLF believed it was naturally latent in everyone but suppressed by society. "In a free society," liberationists declared, "everyone will be gay." They began to urge homosexuals to stop hiding and "come out". The term had been coined by an older generation of homosexuals to describe the act of privately acknowledging one's identity to oneself and other gay people. In a brilliant tactical move, GLF activists transformed it into a public declaration. To come out in Sixties America required deep reservoirs of courage. Anyone who did so risked ostracism and persecution but at least they would naturally wish to ensure the success of the movement. As much as coming out was an act of resistance against a repressive society it was also a declaration of pride in one's self – a sign of liberation. As the movement gained momentum in the Seventies, many ordinary gay men and lesbians came out. Gradually incorporated into society's understanding of what it meant to be gay, the concept "came to represent not simply a single act," as D'Emilio and Freedman note,

> but the adoption of an identity in which the erotic played a central role...No longer merely something you did in bed, sex served to define a mode of living, both private and public, that encompassed a wide range of activities and relationships.

***

Many observers believed the second half of the Sixties constituted a sexual revolution. In some ways they were right. Post-war middle-class Americans had inherited their sexual mores from the inter-war generation, which believed that a good sex life was essential to one's happiness and a successful marriage not because it might lead to children, necessarily, but because it was pleasurable and brought spouses closer together. Of course, sex was to be contained to the conjugal bed, to which, by definition, only heterosexual couples had access. But by the Seventies, as D'Emilio and Freedman argue, this sexual value system threatened to collapse. Consumer capitalism was pushing the erotic beyond the bedroom and plastering it on TV screens, advertisements, books and magazines. Feminists condemned marriage as an oppressive institution while gay liberationists attacked heterosexual

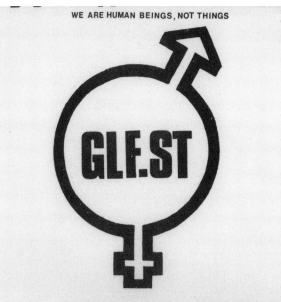

WE ARE HUMAN BEINGS, NOT THINGS

GLF.ST

G.L.F. GAY LIBERATION FRONT   S.T.P. STREET THEATRE PROGRAMME
GAY MEANS HOMOSEXUAL MEANS GOOD

IF YOU DIG IT DO IT

The streets are yours.... make them sing....open out
People like people like you.... come to life.... why
make strangers when you could make friends.... react
respond.... we are now part of your life, become part
of ours....or his....or hers....or theirs....right now.
AND THINK
HOW CAN LOVE CORRUPT, WHEN

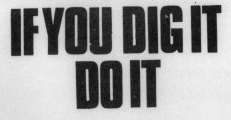

there are as many sexes.... as there are people.

The G.L.F. is fighting for your freedom, as well as ours.
GAY LIBERATION COMES TOGETHER   AT 7.30 p.m. EACH WEDNESDAY AT
THE LONDON SCHOOL OF ECONOMICS
HOUGHTON STREET

A poster advertising the Gay Liberation Front which was formed in 1969 after the Stonewall riots

"supremacy". The only part of this sexual ideology that radicals and capitalists kept was the conviction that sexual pleasure was the key to happiness.

Over the next several decades, this belief would pervade mainstream society, contributing to what D'Emilio and Freedman describe as the "greatest transformation in sexuality" ever experienced by the US. Once one accepted that sex was essential to happiness, how could one justify confining it to marriage? The demographic data from this period suggest that many agreed with this sentiment. From the mid-1960s to the 1980s, Americans married later and were far more likely than their parents to break up (the divorce rate shot up by 90 percent). A growing number of people never got hitched – between 1960 and 1980, the marriage rate declined by a quarter – but that didn't mean that men and women weren't living together. The rate of cohabitation tripled in the Seventies. One long-term analysis of families in Detroit observed that "the decision to marry or remain single is now considered a real and legitimate choice between acceptable alternatives, marking a distinct shift in attitude from that held by Americans in the past." Few expected the singleton to abstain from sex. In the 1950s, less than a quarter of Americans approved of premarital sex for men and women; by the late 1970s, less than a quarter disapproved. As sex permeated the culture, with billboards featuring half-naked Calvin Klein models and album covers flaunting nubile young bodies, teenagers acquired a familiarity with sex and many started having sex at earlier ages.

As sex was being unmoored from marriage, the nature of sex itself was changing. Kinsey encountered few heterosexuals who had experimented with fellatio or cunnilingus; by the 1970s such acts were routinely performed by those in their twenties. Couples were experimenting more and – thanks to the growing use of birth control – having intercourse more often. Couples belonging to earlier generations had disagreed about how often they should have sex; by the Seventies most men and women agreed that they were having the right amount and – at three times a week – relatively high frequencies at that.

The sexual revolution, however, was far from complete. In America its effects were felt far less in rural areas than in cities. The high rate of divorce suggests that many married couples were unhappy. The frequency with which men sexually assaulted women revealed how tentative feminists' progress was. Attacks on gay men and women provided an ugly reminder of the enduring pervasiveness of homophobia.

Many in the West tried to stage a counter-revolution. Unlike the rest of America, religious fundamentalists had held fast to their traditional family values. Like the social purists of the 19th century, they believed that all sex which took place outside of the conjugal bed was sinful. But their Victorian counterparts had not had to contend with sexual radicals who had made significant strides in legislatures and courts, most notably with Roe v Wade, the 1973 Supreme Court ruling which enshrined women's constitutional right to an abortion.

These modern crusaders decided to dive into politics and plotted their counter-attack from within the Republican party. They strove to mobilise the religious right by promising to defeat gay rights, stop the spread of pornography, put an end to school sex-education and restrict abortion. When Ronald Reagan won the presidential election in 1980, political commentators attributed his victory to the support of what would come to be called the religious right. By the 1990s, Republican politicians needed sexual conservatives to win elections.

Over the next three decades, moralists made significant gains in their war with sexual liberals. American evangelicals successfully campaigned to make it ever-more onerous and expensive to get an abortion. By the 1980s, many states were insisting on parental and spousal notifications for abortions. By the following decade, doctors were so frightened of being attacked by violent pro-life forces that 83 percent of American counties did not have a single abortion provider. Between 1985 and 2005, the total number of abortions provided each year fell by 25 percent.

When AIDS struck in the early 1980s, first in the US then quickly spreading to Europe, evangelicals pulled the oldest trick in the book. Echoing Justinian, the sixth-century Eastern Roman Emperor, and Bernardino of Siena, the 15th-century preacher, they declared that the epidemic was divine retribution for sexual deviance. Even more-moderate voices declared that it was time for the sexual revolution to end; in France, respectable publications rejoiced at what they described as a return to chastity. Conservatives' demonisation of homosexuals seemed to work. In 1986, the Supreme Court sustained the constitutionality of state sodomy laws. In 1988, Margaret Thatcher, the prime minister of Britain, passed a law preventing local authorities from "promoting" homosexuality.

Even as latter-day Puritans gained the ears of lawmakers, however, their hold over the public was less certain. As AIDS spread among heterosexuals, public support for homosexuals grew in France and the US. In 1990 President George H. Bush, who was elected with the help of the religious right, signed the Federal Hate Crime Statistics Act, which offered homosexuals some legal protection. With the AIDS epidemic, a trickle of films, TV shows, books and plays about the experiences of lesbian, gay, bisexual, transgender and queer (LGBTQ) people turned into a torrent. Their lives increasingly fascinated the public. When Ellen DeGeneres, a comedian, came out on national television in 1997, she was praised by a large portion of the American public.

By the end of the century, the religious right in the US and conservatives in Europe had become imposing political forces but it was too late to undo the work of their enemies. The lives of most Americans and Europeans followed new rhythms. During the second half of the 20th century, more teenagers had sex with more partners and the age at which they lost their virginity steadily fell. Adults increasingly eschewed lifelong monogamy and heterosexuals made rapid changes to their sexual technique, incorporating oral sex, for instance, into their repertoire. An erotic gender gap persisted: men still orgasmed more often than women, who were largely made responsible for birth control due to widespread use of female contraceptives like the pill. Nonetheless, the changes to the sex lives of late 20th-century Americans and Europeans were profound. Agents of the sexual revolution – entrepreneurs, political radicals, feminists and gay liberationists – had successfully overthrown the conservatism of the 1950s. In the process they loosened the knot tying sexuality to reproduction and gender.

CONCLUSION

As the West rang in the new millennium, a question mark hovered over the sexual revolution: was it here to stay? The signs were promising. Though the media heralded a "post-feminist" age, American legislators were writing feminist sexual politics into their statute books. The Violence Against Women Act (1994), for instance, enacted central planks of the feminists' anti-rape programme by providing funding for states to combat sexual violence against women. While feminism was being institutionalised in the US, LGBTQ activists secured victories in the courts. In 2003, the Supreme Court overturned 500 years of Anglo-American jurisprudence by ruling that state sodomy laws were unconstitutional and, in 2015, that gay couples had the right to marry. In this respect, the Americans were playing catch-up with Western Europe. By 2018, 15 nations had legalised same-sex marriage, among them Germany, France and Great Britain. Undaunted, conservatives remained committed to reversing the changes of the last half century. They met with some success. In 2017 and

2018, the US Senate confirmed Neil Gorsuch and Brett Kavanaugh to the Supreme Court, tipping its balance of power to the right – and prompting rumours that Roe v Wade's days were numbered. Kavanaugh represented a blow for women in another way. His appointment, in spite of the credible allegations of sexual assault levelled against him, revealed the limits of the #MeToo movement, an international campaign to combat sexual harassment and assault which has toppled scores of prominent men around the world since it launched in the US in 2017.

In Europe, new sexually conservative movements, some backed by the Catholic Church, others by secular groups, gained prominence. Violent protests disrupted gay-pride parades in Eastern European cities; in late 2010, right-wing extremists clashed with gay activists in Belgrade. But even as grassroots groups lashed out at sexual progressives, conservative European politicians began to proclaim their devotion to the rights of women and sexual minorities. Anxiety about the influx of Muslim immigrants, characterised as homophobic and misogynistic in the right-wing press, spurred traditionally conservative European political parties to rally round notionally "Western" values. The rise of Islam in Europe had the paradoxical effect of converting many conservative politicians into champions of sexual freedom.

Despite their efforts, conservative King Canutes failed to turn back the tides of change. By the end of the Noughties, growing numbers of Americans postponed marriage until their late 20s or early 30s, if they bothered with matrimony at all – for the first time in 2010, more women weren't living with a husband than were. Sex and family were no longer always mentioned in the same breath as marriage: between 1960 and 2010, the proportion of children born out of wedlock increased eightfold. More and more women decided not to have children at all: the figure doubled between 1970 and 2010. Growing numbers of young people came out as gay, lesbian, bisexual and increasingly, non-binary and transgender. It became possible for Westerners to unmoor sex from gender and reproduction. Though the road to sexual self-determination was bumpy, that was undoubtedly the direction the US was heading in. So was Europe. Broadly speaking, Europeans experienced similar changes to the rhythm of life, though European teenagers were far less likely to become pregnant than American teenagers, thanks to school sex-education programmes.

Though partisans in the political battles over sexuality that had raged in the West in one shape or another for over a century disagreed about whether sexual desire should be liberated or controlled, their arguments shared the same underlying assumption: that sexuality is an important building block of the personality. In the 21st century, scientists characterised it as being shaped by biology, hormones and gender identity. Gay, lesbian and transgender men and women described themselves as "born that way". But as this history has tried to show, the different ways in which sexuality has been defined over millennia show that it is not purely a natural force. Society's conception of sexuality inevitably shapes our behaviour and our understanding of ourselves as sexual beings.

FURTHER READING

The indispensable guide to the history of sexuality in Europe is Anna Clark's *Desire* (2008). Its history in America is best told by John D'Emilio and Estelle B. Freedman in *Intimate Matters* (2018 edn). In *Histories of Sexuality: Antiquity to Sexual Revolution* (2004), Stephen Garton provides a thorough overview of the discipline's historiography and the lively theoretical debates concerning the nature of past sexualities. In contrast to these academic works, Eric Berkowitz's *Sex and Punishment* (2013), is a rollicking exploration of the various means by which the powerful have regulated sex over the last 4,000 years, and is stocked full of delicious tidbits. Below is a brief list for further reading. The place of publication is London unless otherwise stated.

Bray, Alan. *Homosexuality in Renaissance England* (1982)
Brown, Peter. *The Body and Society: Men, Women, and Sexual Renunciation in Early Christianity* (New York, 2008 edn)
Chauncey, George. *Gay New York: Gender, Urban Culture and the Making of the Gay Male World 1890-1940* (New York, 1994)
Cook, Hera. *The Long Sexual Revolution: English Women, Sex, and Contraception 1800-1975* (Oxford, 2004)
Cook, Matt. *London and the Culture of Homosexuality, 1885-1914* (Cambridge, 2003)
Dabhoiwala, Faramerz. *The Origins of Sex: A History of the First Sexual Revolution* (2012)
Foucault, Michel. *The History of Sexuality* (1985)
Harper, Kyle. *From Sin to Shame: The Christian Transformation of Sexual Morality in Late Antiquity* (2013)
Herzog, Dagmar. *Sexuality in Europe: A Twentieth-Century History* (Cam-

bridge, 2011)

ed. Hunt, Lynn. *The Invention of Pornography: Obscenity and the Origins of Modernity, 1500-1800* (New York, 1993)

Karras, Ruth Mazo. *Sexuality in Medieval Europe: Doing Unto Others* (New York, 2017)

Laqueur, Thomas. *Making Sex: Body and Gender from the Greeks to Freud* (1990)

McLaren, Angus. *Twentieth-Century Sexuality: A History* (Oxford, 1999)

ed. Nye, Robert A. Sexuality (Oxford, 1999)

Oosterhuis, Harry. *Stepchildren of Nature: Psychiatry and the Making of Sexual Identity* (Chicago, 2000)

Ormand, Kirk. *Controlling Desires: Sexuality in Ancient Greece and Rome* (Austin, 2018 edn)

Richards, Jeffrey. *Sex, Dissidence and Damnation: Minority Groups in the Middle Ages* (London, 1990)

Rocke, Michael. *Forbidden Friendships: Homosexuality and Male Culture in Renaissance Florence* (Oxford, 1996)

Stone, Lawrence. *The Family, Sex and Marriage in England 1500-1800* (1979 edn)

Weeks, Jeffrey. *Sex, Politics and Society: The Regulation of Sexuality Since 1800* (2018 edn)

Wiesner-Hanks, Merry E. *Christianity and Sexuality in the Early Modern World* (2000)

INDEX